Decision Making and Healthcare Management for Frontline Staff

Decision Making and Healthcare Management for Frontline Staff

RUSSELL GURBUTT

Foreword by
Pat Donovan

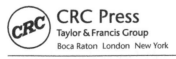

CRC Press
Taylor & Francis Group
Boca Raton London New York

CRC Press is an imprint of the
Taylor & Francis Group, an **informa** business

First published 2011 by Radcliffe Publishing

Published 2016 by CRC Press
Taylor & Francis Group
6000 Broken Sound Parkway NW, Suite 300
Boca Raton, FL 33487-2742

CRC Press is an imprint of Taylor & Francis Group, an Informa business

No claim to original U.S. Government works

ISBN-13: 978-1-84619-048-3 (pbk)

British Library Cataloguing in Publication Data

A catalogue record for this book is available from the British Library.

Typeset by KnowledgeWorks Global Ltd, Chennai, India

DECISION MAKING AND HEALTHCARE MANAGEMENT
FOR FRONTLINE STAFF

Care worker to a porter: *Management don't have a clue about what we do.*

* * *

Health service report: *Our staff is our greatest asset.*

* * *

Ward staff nurse to researcher: *The sister should be in the office doing her stuff.*
Researcher: *What sort of things does she do then?*
Staff nurse: *Well I'm not too sure but she should leave us to get on with the clinical care. She has a lot of paperwork and meetings and things like that.*

* * *

Ward round doctor to staff nurse: *Where is the Sister for the ward round?*
Staff nurse: *I have been looking after this team so I'll do the round with you.*
Doctor: *I'll come back later when the sister is around.*

* * *

Relative making a telephone enquiry to the ward: *Is the sister available?*
Staff nurse: *She's busy at the moment, can I help you?*
Relative: *No I'll wait for the sister.*
Relative (some time later): *Sister, could you tell me what the ward visiting times are?*

* * *

Health informatician: *Computers and the e-record will really make a difference.*

* * *

Service user: *There's a lot of money wasted in the NHS – and it doesn't need to be.*

* * *

Consultant: *I'm sorry you've waited so long, we usually overrun in clinic.*

* * *

Unit manager to staff group: *There will be a freeze on all new recruitment until further notice. Advise me on what you think the implications will be over the next six months for your service.*

* * *

Chief executive to senior managers: *The economic situation requires us to make a saving of half a million pounds across the service this year in addition to the same amount already saved this year. Tell me how you propose to achieve that without compromising service delivery?*

* * *

Does that sound familiar and does it have to be like this?

Contents

Foreword

Not another book on management you cry. This is not *just* another book. Russell Gurbutt has managed in this short book to look at health service management from a multitude of perspectives in an original and creative way. This is not a stuffy text book, but is written in a very personal style to the reader. He uses letter writing in an innovative way which allows Russell to incorporate personal reflection on experience which gives vision to words. As stated, Russell has 'translated ideas and visions into practice' in this book. Because of the personal writing style there is clear explanation and application of theoretical concepts throughout, and this application of theory is grounded in the practice that is depicted in the text. Interactive participation is encouraged and clearly guided. Even though the approach is via letter writing there is no 'talking down' to the reader but a critical approach is used which is always respectful and challenging. It is good to see sense being made of theoretical concepts and managerial speak, as well as criticisms of that managerial speak. Although in many ways this work is grounded within the UK experience there is a lot that can be taken for alternative healthcare services. Russell takes the reader not only around the hospital but also over mountains and into caves, demonstrating his wide and varied life experience which he uses to full advantage. The model used also takes into account the context of the practice and this is what is not seen in many other management books. I recommend this book to all health professionals, whether at the beginning of their career (very like Marie in the book) or those who need a fresh insight into their own managerial position, as well as educators who may want to use the coffee break exercises with their students. I will certainly be advising my Masters students to use this as part of their exploration of health service management.

Pat Donovan
Principal Lecturer and Lead Midwife for Education
University of Central Lancashire
October 2010

Preface

Healthcare delivery is a busy, complex activity involving numerous people and resources. Those who work on the frontline in this sector can find their focus narrowed down to the immediate local context at the expense of engagement with many issues that impact on the wider service. Even within the local context there are many issues to contend with, and making sense of how these are integrated into the wider service can seem confusing or impossible. However, neglecting engagement with the wider healthcare organisation renders the frontline practitioner vulnerable to being reactive to external pressures. Whilst this might be the reality of frontline experience, it is not an ideal situation, especially in the context of a continually changing environment that is typical of modern services.

I kept this problem in mind when writing this book that seeks to assist frontline staff in making sense of their complex world. In this book I have set out to use a series of reference points to prompt thought and exploration. Through correspondence between a lecturer and a practitioner, a descriptive model of the clinical landscape (topography) of the workplace that seeks to render it understandable is developed. This is used as a reference to facilitate enquiry. The purpose of the dialogue is not to expound detailed theoretical accounts of organisational design and policy, but to pose a series of triggers for the reader to consider in relation to their own clinical situation. What is done in clinical work is based on what we know, with the decision making process being shaped by the participants and their environments. It is necessary, therefore, to appreciate these contexts so as to be aware of factors that shape decision making.

Skilled decision making is essential amongst service delivery staff so that they can be effective agents of change rather than simply reacting to externally-imposed change. Success in this regard relies on information, and the model outlined in this book provides reference points to determine where information is needed and used to think through change and its wider implications for service delivery. This is not an aimless exploration taking in the theoretical 'sights' so to speak, but rather a purposeful journey that should cause the reader to reflect on personal learning in relation to their role.

For educators, this book also provides a different type of reader around which care management modules, teaching and learning can be designed. The model has been used in teaching a range of clinical staff, such as nursing students, registered nurses and experienced doctors. It has been used to stimulate discussion and critical analysis of roles, processes and purpose, together with an appreciation of factors in health service delivery beyond the individual staff's immediate professional interests.

If you are not directly involved in clinical delivery, this book might assist you in seeing the service through different eyes. Fresh insights into the complex clinical landscape are valuable to promote the importance of service users at the heart of the system. Healthcare service design must always promote a focus on service users rather than take precedence over them; it is therefore essential to recognise factors shaping service decision making that might shift this focus. By paying attention to the wider picture, a healthcare worker whatever their role, can learn to recognise and influence decisions across the entire clinical landscape.

Russell Gurbutt, Preston

About the author

Dr Russell Gurbutt had a military background and, following active service, moved to healthcare work in 1984 and, more recently, has worked in higher education. Professional work has ranged across public, private and voluntary sectors, and has included providing healthcare consultancy services. Current work continues in the arena of wisdom and decision making, and might be summarised as follows: 'A wise teacher's words spur students into action and emphasize important truths. The collected sayings of the wise are like guidance from a shepherd. But my child be warned: There is no end of opinions ready to be expressed. Studying them can go on forever and can become very exhausting! Here is my conclusion: Fear God and obey his commands, for this is the duty of every person.' (Ecclesiastes 12: 11-13 NLT)

To Dawne, Jessica & Thomas

A guide to using this book

Let me now proceed to introduce Professor Cartmel, who is corresponding as an informal mentor with a former nursing student following her appointment to a new management role. The book is organised in sections, each of which is a cluster of letters. Each letter is followed by a coffee break reflection or activity designed to develop further exploration of the subject.

Decision making and the big picture: making sense of health service delivery

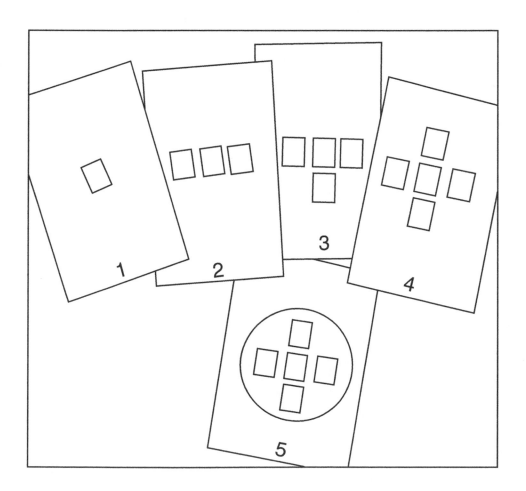

Tom Cartmel, a nursing professor, was taking a sabbatical year in the Netherlands. During this period he struck up a correspondence with Marie, one of his former students. Her recent clinical appointment and associated professional studies had opened up new lines of enquiry, particularly about health service delivery and decision making. His initial reply (that subsequently developed into a regular correspondence) focused on the relationship between people at the heart of health service management. He continued....

LETTER 1:   THE MAIN FOCUS

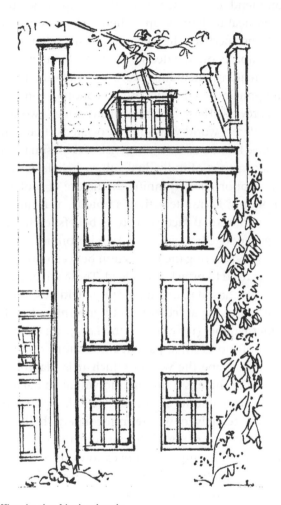

IMAGE 1   At an office in the Netherlands

Dear Marie,

Thank you for your recent letter. It was good to hear how you are progressing in your new clinical role, and how this has spurred you onto consider wider aspects of health service delivery and related decision making.

As you are well aware, to participate in health service delivery is to move into a complex world where even the briefest of clinical interactions is the collision of two distinct worlds. One is a professional world employing particular knowledge and skills applied to assessment, planning, intervention and evaluation. The other is the service user's (or patient's) world. Each world shares common human spiritual, physical, social and psychological characteristics.

At their intersection the participants bring something unique to clinical decision making. One observes, listens and even empathises whilst considering the clinical action to recommend and pursue. The other's experience of their own stable, improving or failing health status shapes their negotiation and accommodation of the professional's perspective. The dynamic of this relationship shapes mutual understanding and impacts on any decisions made. Many factors influence a professional's decision making, including practice standards, professional conduct, political healthcare policies, legal boundaries, economic constraints, employment obligations and peer review. These frame the professional's world-view, whereas the patient may hold a different world-view (and associated different health beliefs) that forms their interpretive framework to make sense of their situation. This interpretive framework can be a construct of individual values, beliefs, knowledge (that might challenge some assumptions underpinning the nature of professional knowledge) and notions of autonomy. Each interaction is unique, as is the relative importance afforded to different contextual factors such as beliefs, cultural practices, gender, education and language together with social and economic differences. Whilst at the moment I'm only considering the interaction between two people, between two worlds wider contexts need to be acknowledged. These include the setting (perhaps a clinic, a walk-in centre, hospital, a refugee camp, field hospital or the individual's home), and socio-political (a particular society, government and laws), geographical, regional and international (for example the European Union) contexts.

Thus, the briefest of professional-patient interactions occurs within a series of bounding contexts that shape the way in which it is played out. It follows that within this commonality there is a unique individual characteristic to healthcare provision – it is not amenable to a 'one size fits all' approach. However, when considering health service delivery we are immediately challenged with a tension between providing services for many whilst ensuring these are tailored to the needs of the individual. When this emphasis moves towards a service for many it can render the individual as an object to be processed. You will be familiar with often heard descriptions like 'another hip replacement', an 'elective surgical case' the 'appendicectomy in bed three'. This is no more than the patient seen as an object and indicates a shift has occurred from a person- to process-centred approach to healthcare delivery.

The challenge is clear Marie: we want to promote health service delivery focused on individuals, not categories or cases. The tensions inherent in managing, balancing and resolving multiple pressures and responses to short-term issues of the day can deflect from this focus. Thus, the decisions that you will make as a health service worker or manager will have to recognise the pervading complexity but preserve a service-user focus.

(In her letter Marie had hinted that the halcyon days as a student with limited clinical accountability and responsibility were long gone. Now she was moving on from the basics of professional practice to a greater involvement in care management. Professor Cartmel considered her question: *'How do I make sense of this in an understandable way? Where do I start?'*) He took up this question…

Marie, if we can agree on the focus of service provision we are ready to understand how a complex service can be arrayed around a service user.

(Cartmel had some suggestions to guide her knowledge and experience development pathway. He knew that the analogy of an iceberg was relevant to understanding how some staff perceived health service delivery. They only saw a fraction of it from their location, namely the ice protruding above the water's surface whilst remaining largely unaware of the extent of submerged berg.)

If we apply an iceberg analogy to service design in which most of the berg or service is unseen, those who only make decisions on what is seen have a limited appreciation of how the system operates. Working with what is seen rather than including the unseen generates a knowledge gap that renders them 'organisationally blind' – we need to see the whole. This conveniently returns to my opening sentences about the context of the intersection of distinct professional and service-user worlds – it would be a useful step to examine and explain the organisational structure of your service as a whole so as to appreciate the immediate context of your decision making.

Kind regards,

Yours,

Cartmel

Coffee break: organisational design

Spend some time exploring and reflecting on the design of your local organisation.

- Examine and describe the organisational design of your local service – what do you think comprises its constituent parts, and how are these arranged and interrelated?

- How would you represent it as a diagram? (When making sense of complex situations it can help to sketch out different ways in which constituent parts can be represented in relation to each other.)

- Does the arrangement that you have sketched have a particular shape, and does this have any significance in representing where service delivery decisions are made and how they are supported? Is there an 'official' representation of the shape of your healthcare organisation? If it differs from your initial sketch does this raise any challenges to your account of where service delivery decisions are made and how they are supported?

LETTER 2: REPRESENTING HEALTH SERVICE COMPLEXITY – THE BIG PICTURE

Dear Marie,

Thanks for your swift response – I agree that it seems as if there are lots of jigsaw pieces but no overall picture to decide how they should all fit together, or to even know if we have all of the pieces in our possession. So to help you I will describe a big picture, one that will serve as a reference to locate and arrange the constituent parts, and will use it to navigate around the complex world of healthcare delivery. One advantage of this is to avoid a parochial view that is merely concerned with local issues and partisan professional interests. Furthermore, it will support a central focus on the service user.

Whilst I accept that all models reduce real world complexity, they bring into focus different service elements and their interrelatedness. Once identified, these elements can be explored in relation to decision making. After reading this you might consider that the model needs developing – feel free to do so, it is merely a tool to assist your understanding of the whole. This model, which I will describe next, has five principal elements of which the central one is front-line service delivery.

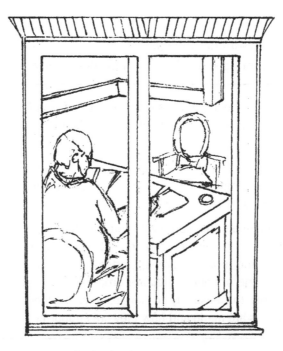

IMAGE 2 From an office in the Netherlands

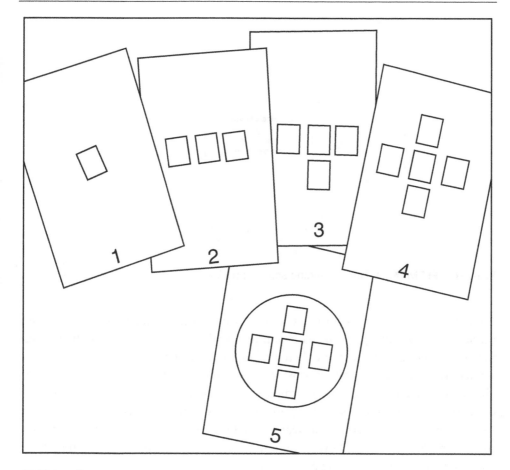

IMAGE 3 Sketching out a model

(Taking some leaves of cartridge paper from his folio he began sketching the model, or as he labelled it a 'big picture', to include in the letter.)

Element 1 concerns service delivery that lies at the heart of any healthcare organisation. Healthcare should focus on the service user's needs. Often they are thought of as patients, implying a relationship between the individual and the organisation based on an illness model. However, such a model might not be appropriate as a service can embrace a health perspective where people access it for reasons other than diagnosis and treatment – hence employing the label 'service user' avoids the medical (illness) model association and offers scope for a different user – provider relationship.

The place of service delivery is varied, but wherever that is care needs to be delivered in a safe environment with safe processes. This requires robust governance arrangements that address a range of legal, regulatory, professional, policy and economic factors.

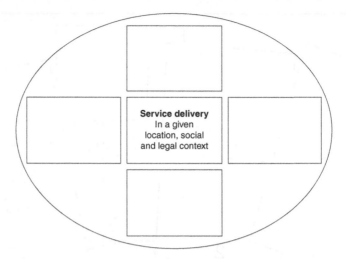

FIGURE 1 ELEMENT 1 Understanding service provision

Element 2 directs attention onto the trajectory of the service user as they access services from within a particular community, use the service and ultimately progress to some other destination, possibly returning to the host community. It follows that service delivery needs to be responsive to demand, and this requires information about its level and nature. This is termed health intelligence and involves a methodology used to assess the designated population's healthcare needs. Furthermore, any measurement of need requires a clear understanding of what exactly is understood by the term 'health' – this, however, is a movable feast, and there are different views about health and the meaning of being healthy.

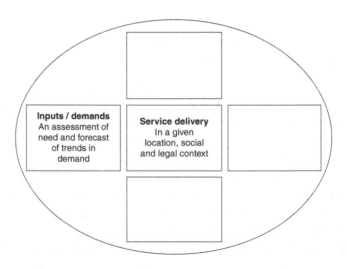

FIGURE 2 ELEMENT 2 Service demands

Element 3 continues the theme of a service user trajectory or journey, and directs attention towards the endpoint of exiting the service. At this stage questions are asked about service delivery processes and their outcomes. These might include: What was the experience of service provision along the service user trajectory? Did service provision achieve its goals for the particular service user? To what extent did provision match demand? Information analysis at this juncture facilitates the generation of findings and conclusions about service quality, effectiveness and efficiency. Naturally, this analysis is no mere paper exercise – the information is used in decision making about provision, processes, resources, quality enhancement and strategic direction. All service delivery requires resources which are the focus of the next element.

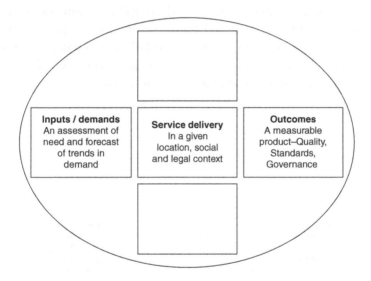

FIGURE 3 ELEMENT 3 Service outcomes

Element 4 represents service resources and highlights that nothing occurs along the service user trajectory without them. Even a voluntary service requires resources (such as a place, people, time and possibly equipment). When I speak of resources I'm referring to financial, physical, human, and information.

Financial resources – the service has to be paid for from somewhere. The funding can come from charity, the service user, an insurance scheme or public taxation (or a combination of these). Without resources nothing happens (as some English NHS Trusts demonstrated in 2007 when they addressed local financial deficits by unit closures and staff redundancies). A business plan should underpin resource management.

Financial resources enable staff to provide services – healthcare delivery is essentially a social organisation combining the efforts of a multidisciplinary workforce.

Resource management determines the mix of staff with defined levels of expertise to deliver the service as planned. It also necessitates understanding of the intellectual resources of the staff team, their knowledge and experience that is often forgotten when plans are made to alter staffing teams, skill mixes and establishment levels.

Service delivery involves the utilisation of physical technological resources (equipment and supplies), along with associated processes of procurement, monitoring, use and disposal. These too must be managed to ensure safe usage, be it a syringe, suction machine or bed.

Information is necessary to support management of the service user through the trajectory of service delivery. Effective service delivery needs quality information – about all aspects of the service – such as the assessments of demand, delivery processes, resource usage, workforce development and outcomes of completed episodes of care. Information requires governance, including data organization, quality, generation, storage, security, retrieval and transmission along approved communication channels. Each element cannot exist in isolation, and has to be directed and coordinated through careful information management. This gives rise to a need for an executive strategic management and leadership element.

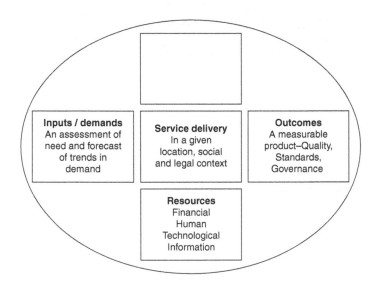

FIGURE 4 ELEMENT 4 Service resources

Element 5 of the service model distinguishes between current day to day operations and the direction of where and what the service will be in the future. Strategic planning and leadership occupies this part of the model. Local operational management has to harmonise with the corporate direction of the whole organisation. To permit otherwise would create tensions and fractures that would adversely impact on other parts of the service. Given that independent development is incompatible with a focused corporate direction there is a need for an integrated and coordinated strategic management function. This draws on the organization of information to be able to lead, direct and evaluate the whole service operation so that it performs in accordance with its own plans, goals and contracts of service provision. There is also an external function of horizon scanning the external environment to monitor and develop strategic responses to external trends. When combined, these two functions (strategic management and leadership) facilitate decision making about enhancing the internal organisational operations, their development or redesign to make them fit for purpose to meet externally changing patterns of demand.

As I draw this letter to a close I need to distinguish between leadership and management. Both are required in health service delivery and an individual can combine both, placing different emphasis on these roles according to the situation at a given time.

If I use the analogy of a machine, the manager has a responsibility to ensure that the 'mechanism' runs smoothly and efficiently. They don't tinker with the machine or reorganise its cogs and levers. They just ensure that it operates as designed. They only intervene in the machine to restore a failure in its operation. The leader on the other hand makes decisions about the way in which the machine works, asks if it needs redesigning or even if it is the right machine at all to make the required product? Both roles can be fulfilling and both are necessary.

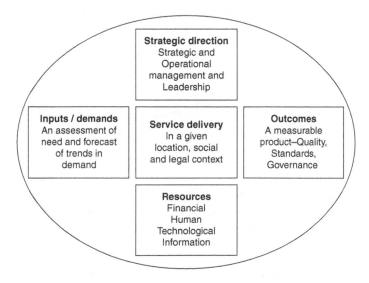

FIGURE 5 ELEMENT 5 Strategic direction and overall bounding context

I began by claiming that this model, a big picture of the service's constituent parts, will facilitate your navigation around the complex world of healthcare delivery. But there is one further addition to note because this service does not exist in a vacuum.

A circle drawn around the model denotes the context of a local organisation within a particular region and country. This bounding circle alerts you to remember that everything can be understood within contexts – local, national and international. Whatever exists in the external environment impacts on the organization's internal working.

When you hear sayings such as the 'signs of the times' and 'the writing is on the wall' or 'reform is needed' these indicate an interpretation of the context. This implies that someone has the skills to interpret these signs to inform decision making. To be an effective manager and leader you need to take a big picture perspective as the context of your decision making. This will aid identification of information requirements to support decision making relating to the service as a whole. Unilateral decision making made about an aspect of delivery (the central element in the model) without appreciating its impact on all of the other elements is unlikely to be successful or sustainable. Furthermore, your decisions need to demonstrate awareness of the 'shifting sands' of the wider context than just local operations.

Well Marie, now that I have explained the model, the big picture, I suggest that you revisit your original sketch of organisational design and see to what extent this offers a logical shape for all of the constituent parts that you successfully identified. Explore the executive element of your local organisation further to see if you can locate an account expressing why the organisation exists and where it is heading, after all, your future career is bound up with this whilst you work there.

Kind regards,
Cartmel

Coffee break: models, purpose, mission and vision

Here are some questions to help develop your initial exploration of your local organisation.

- Use the model as a route map and determine the extent to which it helps to explain the local organisation. What fits? Where does it fit? What else can you add within the elements of the model? Can you see any new elements emerging?

- What is the explicit purpose of your chosen local healthcare organisation?

- What, if any, is the published mission and vision?

LETTER 3:   PURPOSE – MISSION AND VISION

Dear Marie,

Thanks for responding so quickly – so you found it helpful, and I agree that drawing diagrams is a useful tool in making sense of a busy and complex environment.

I liked your account of the 'purpose' and as I suspected you noticed that there seemed to be more than one organisational purpose. Whilst it is convenient to draft fine sounding statements about the organisation existing to serve and provide person-centred services, this is not always the lived experience. In military aviation the ground crew organisation exists to enable the pilot to fly a serviceable and fit for purpose aeroplane. Similarly, everything in a health service should exist to support the delivery of patient-centered services. You might represent this as a pyramid with the pinnacle as the purpose of the organisation, or a circle with the service user in the centre. An example follows (from the NHS) highlighting the centrality of the service user, which in this case casts them as a patient-customer:

> 'There is still much to do and with the developments included in this plan we have a real desire to continue to improve the patient experience of our services. We recognise the importance of a customer focus and that the manner in which our excellent clinical services are provided in terms of convenience, communication style and respect are important to our patients and their families.'[1]

But is it like this in reality? The fact that statements need to be made about person-centered services implies that the focus can shift elsewhere. Some decades ago I observed how in a former asylum the rigid routines of meals, baths, drug rounds, required clothing, and the timing of lights on and lights off subsumed patient individuality and choice. Years later I encountered a similar situation when taking up a new ward management post. Curiously enough I recently came across a care worker who had changed a minor routine in a care home to make a working pattern better for the residents. That well-meaning action caused uproar within the staff team as the routine had been established by someone who had ceased employment over two years previously and it was seemingly 'set in stone' even though it had outlived its useful purpose. That event illustrated the potency of routines and resistance that deflects the focus from providing patient-centered services. You will recall in a previous letter I remarked that some staff were 'organisationally blind', and in this case the carers needed to stand aside from their routines so as to be able to look afresh at them. Time doesn't change things – but action by thoughtful people can.

The focus can change for a variety of reasons and a way of detecting this is helped by the words of an Anglican confession[2] in which we acknowledge that we err 'by negligence, by weakness and by our own deliberate fault'. As with a confession and repentance (a wilful change of direction) management decision making requires a realistic appraisal of the situation as a precursor to change followed by an action plan. Such appraisals can be made against the stated organisational purpose. These are readily found on the organisation's web pages, for example:

'The Trust's principal purpose is to serve the community by the provision of goods and services for the purposes of healthcare.'[3]

Other organisations express this as function:

The function of the Trust is to provide goods and services, including education and training, research, accommodation and other facilities, for purposes related to the provision of healthcare, subject to any restriction in the authorization.[4]

Notice how the purpose of healthcare provision is focused on patients:

We will: Put patients first, Take pride in what we do, Respect others, Strive to be the best, Act with integrity.[5]

It is helpful when the purpose or mission is underpinned by explicit values and given clear strategic direction as in the example of this New York State Hospital.[6]

Our Mission: Our mission is to care compassionately for those we serve with dedication to excellence and Christian ideals.

Our Values: Service of the Poor, Reverence, Integrity, Wisdom, Creativity, Dedication

Our Vision: St. Mary's Hospital at Amsterdam will be a strong Catholic regional hospital dedicated to improving the health of the entire community with special attention to the poor and underserved. Patients, physicians and associates will prefer us because of our reputation for excellence and service, and our commitment to safety and quality.

Notice how some organisations' values feature more prominently in the public domain. The Toronto Mount Sinai Hospital[7] elaborates on the detail of these within their mission, vision and values statement:

Our Vision: To deliver and model world-class healthcare, translating research and education into excellent patient care in the programs we offer.

Our Mission: Mount Sinai Hospital is dedicated to discovering and delivering the best patient care with the heart and values true to our heritage.

Our Values: Our fundamental values allow us to serve our patients effectively and distinguish Mount Sinai Hospital and the Samuel Lunenfeld Research Institute as a model healthcare centre.

These values include:

> **Excellence:** Pursuing excellence and innovation in everything we do. Our ideas and enthusiasm help us continuously improve.
>
> **Service:** Providing patient and family-focused care that is sensitive to our multi-cultural community.
>
> **Teamwork:** Taking a collaborative and multidisciplinary team approach to patient care, teaching and research.
>
> **Collaboration:** Creating dynamic partnerships both internally and externally to benefit patients and our role as a teaching hospital.
>
> **Respect and Diversity:** Valuing and respecting each other's differences.
>
> **Leadership:** Promoting the development and growth of leaders at all levels through continuous learning and knowledge sharing.

When using the confession formula applied to vision, mission and values it can be seen that vision is the belief of where we can be, mission is the behaviour required to achieve the vision and values are the guiding principles that direct behaviour. The acid test is how statements on paper translate into service delivery. What do you think?

Yours,
Cartmel

Coffee break: purpose, mission and vision translated into practice

Take time to consider how statements of purpose, mission, vision and values translate into the real world practice of service delivery.

> - What leads the workforce to live the values? (Many role descriptions require applicants to support and uphold the organisation's values; others require staff to live their values.)
> - How can an organisation ensure that its values are supported?
> - To what extent do the values of the employing organization match your values?
> - If values differ do compromises need to be made that cause conflicts of conscience?
> - In what ways does labelling a service user as a patient or customer reflect the perspective of the organisation?

LETTER 4: PURPOSE, MISSION, VISION AND OWNERSHIP

Dear Marie,

It is true to say that people are the means of translating ideas and visions into practice, but they need to utilise the structures available to facilitate this process. These can be formal or informal structures. Furthermore, when embedding a vision throughout the organisation it is advantageous if there has been wide consultation to engender ownership amongst each part, whether it involves staff in a mobile unit, a ward, a surgery, a clinic, a store or a maintenance department.

Shared vision development also happens in other settings, such as amongst education providers, and can take up to a year to complete as a process of listening to staff and other stakeholders is worked through. When this process is circumvented and a smaller group forges the vision there is a greater selling job to be done as it will not necessarily be immediately understood (as the process of discussion has excluded some) and will be interpreted in different ways (as the checking of the wording of final drafts has not been open to wider review).

The launch of a vision can be via a formal, staged event – a launch day and briefings. Formal channels are used to communicate a vision, including staff briefings, staff meetings, video podcasts and bulletins attached to wage slips as well as staff development events and away days. A vision often has symbols of corporate identity such as a logo, a strap line, a uniform, literature, pens and publications. Alignment to the vision is termed 'being on message' – a contemporary term for 'singing from the same hymn sheet'. To be 'off message', however, is to signal a different direction that potentially threatens the organisation. Division is counterproductive to harmonising resources to achieve the vision.

I've witnessed resistance where some staff groups in front-line service delivery continued to do their 'own thing' despite a published vision and mission. To some extent it demonstrated a failure to embed the vision and deliver real change in practice. In such circumstances there is a lot of work to be undertaken to assert leadership and vision, and to challenge conflicting practice.

How convenient it might seem to have staff as round pegs in round holes as the required people for the required jobs. Life is more complex, and individuals should be expected to think and their views should be worth listening to. That doesn't oblige you to act on their views, but it is helpful to let people have their say as long as that is undertaken in a constructive and not a divisive way. But not every manager wants to work with the existing staff group and instead they seek to build a new team around them that will ensure delivery of a new vision. This entails shedding staff deemed not to fit the renewed organisation. Sometimes they are referred to as 'old money', having worked under a previous leadership, and their practices and perspectives are now judged as incompatible with current requirements. This is sometimes seen when an executive leadership changes and new staff are employed whilst others have their contracts terminated (often through a process of having to reapply for their jobs in an open competition).

However, even if you skillfully sell a vision it will not stop staff and volunteers making their own judgements about it and the implications for their practice. Their conclusions can lead to resistance to change. Some staff might leave as they indicate their lack of ownership by 'voting with their feet' whilst others can form a counter-culture that creates tensions and frustrates development.

In terms of decision making we need to consider first where we stand in relation to vision, mission, purpose and values, and decide the extent to which we own them. In one job spanning a decade I observed that the vision altered three times, and each time was presented in a new and exciting way (to obscure the fact that the anticipated strategic plan had failed). Unsurprisingly, staff noticed the continuity of core business amidst change in statements made by the executive. There was a suspicion that such statements would change again and raised a question whether there could be ownership of care delivery alongside selective disregard of some or all of the existing vision statement.

Having identified our position and ownership in relation to the vision, identify the formal channels through which it is communicated. Having completed that you can consider the extent to which the vision is owned in your local workplace associated with interpretation of the vision statement, its communication and ownership. A useful technique is to use the confessional framework about actions that should have been taken to engender ownership but were not afforded sufficient priority (negligence), steps that should have been taken but potent forces have shaped some other less effective action (weakness) and steps that were deliberately taken that have not engendered ownership (wilful act). In this way you can reflect and expand your insight into measures that promote stakeholder ownership or disinvestment.

I wonder what the situation is in your workplace?

Yours truly,
Cartmel

Coffee break: promoting ownership
Take time to explore ways in which ownership is achieved in your local workplace.

- Look around your local unit and reflect on what you hear and observe regarding vision, and ask 'does this promote ownership or not?'
- What methods are used to communicate and translate vision into practice?
- Vision and ownership – to what extent does being 'off message' challenge the local organisation?
- What organisational response does being 'off message' generate?
- When can being 'off message' be healthy?
- What does an organisation lose when it seeks to shed staff who previously worked under a different executive and vision?

LETTER 5:   SHIFTING FOCUS

Dear Marie,

Thanks for writing – it's raining and cold but hopefully not where you are. In reading your reflections on ownership I was particularly struck by the incidental comment about a shifting focus in service delivery. This can occur even with the best of intentions as the influence of different stakeholders and drivers for change come to bear on decision making. It also can lead staff to question the organisation's purpose. Recently I came across this with a healthcare provider that prided itself on its care for people who suffered life-limiting disease. When its long term-business plan was published based on an increase in hours of care over a set number of years this was interpreted by some staff as a meaningless figure. They questioned how many hours they currently delivered and what difference the new target figure would make to their service. Furthermore, some understood it as a reduction in quality in favour of increased workload volume that privileged economics over beneficiaries of the service.

In terms of decision making, whenever there is incomplete ownership of vision, scope exists for competing voices to challenge and set a different agenda. A vacuum always leads to tension that must be recognised and managed. Some private companies can be autocratic – you accept the way of working and become a company person or move on. Public sector organisations can be more democratic, and facilitate staff consultation and contribution. What matters is to understand the ground rules of how the local organisation works (some of which will be explicit in policies and procedures), and how its vision and purpose are shaped. Then you will be better placed to understand how the intended purpose might have shifted (through executive direction) or might be interpreted as having shifted (through the way in which it was communicated to staff).

Recalling a point in a previous letter there is also a focus to consider at the interface between professional and service user where decision making can be service-user led, collaborative, shared, or professionally led. Any oscillation along this continuum will privilege one participant's views over the other. So when a service user is labeled as a patient there is corresponding support for a professional viewpoint that makes it easier to shift the focus of decision making towards their own interests that will in some measure be at the expense of the patient's autonomy.

So clarity of focus is important – people need to be clear about the vision and purpose of the organization they are working for otherwise a time will come when the difference in what they think this is and what it actually is will cause tension. Furthermore, given that decisions are shaped by multiple stakeholders we need to understand who these are as part of understanding why organisational focus might shift.

The rain is easing and the sky is breaking – tomorrow will be a brighter day. Use your study time to check out which stakeholders shape the focus of your local healthcare organisation.

Yours truly,
Cartmel

Coffee break: identifying stakeholders

Consider the organisational model and each of its elements to determine who the stakeholders are.

- Who are the stakeholders within each element?

- Who are the stakeholders outside of the organisation?

- Are some more influential than others? If so, why?

LETTER 6: WHOSE SERVICE IS IT? – STAKEHOLDERS

Dear Marie,

It's not unreasonable to think that national government is a major stakeholder with responsibility for, and control of health services, especially if it claims to be a national service. In England, for example, the National Health Service is led and 'safeguarded' by the elected government for the benefit of the whole population. This view is evident in publications such as The NHS Improvement Plan[1] in which the government's agenda (via the Department of Health) is to 'put people at the heart of public services'. Its stake in policy implementation further highlights its role in determining the types of services required both now and in the future. In an excerpt from its operating framework[2] economics, reform and selected service priorities constitute the government's stakeholder focus.

The NHS is, and will remain, committed to delivering the plans set out in National Standards, Local Action, published in July 2004, covering the three years 2005/6 to 2007/8. Nationally, we shall be putting a particular focus in 2006/7 on:
- achieving robust financial health;
- pushing forward the implementation of reform; and
- achieving six specific service priorities derived from the Planning and Priorities Framework.

Support for this view is linked to a service-user perspective ('what you told us' and 'what we are doing'), thus affording the government credibility as advocates for the public. In this they outlined how:

> *'Our health, our care, our say: a new direction for community services* set out a new and ambitious vision for the future of our community services, responding to what people want and expect of services in the 21st century. In the consultation and debates that preceded the White Paper, they told us very clearly what they are looking for: seamless health and social care to support them to stay healthy and to lead independent lives; more services provided locally; and services that are fair to all, with more help for the people who need them most.'

Notice how stakeholder actions were linked to public demand and changing patterns of need:

> This shift is necessary, not only because it responds to what people want, but also because the needs of today's and tomorrow's users of health and social care services are very different from those of yesterday.

However, we need to adopt a critical stance when evaluating any stakeholder perspective. The problem with the government's claim is that it implies that they possess the definitive evidence on the nature of needs and the interpretation of patterns of change. Given that their consultation was based on 140 000 respondents (out of a population over 60 million), at the very least we need to know the profile of the sample and the questions that they were asked. You already know that this is open to scrutiny as competing political groups hold different ideological positions on the role of the state in public health, the economics of healthcare and priority setting.

We can move on to sketch a stakeholder diagram using the model. Internal stakeholders are located in the boxes representing elements of healthcare delivery and the bounding circle distinguishes those located outside of the local organisation. A judgement can be made about the relative influence of stakeholders and factors that cause this to wax or wane.

Tensions, collaboration and conflict may exist between the internal stakeholders as they seek to assert their influence over their 'domain' and privilege their view wherever their purpose is served or perceived to be threatened.

Internal stakeholder groups are not a cohesive whole as might be suggested in organisational diagrams. Service users as stakeholders are often aligned to diagnosis groups – the MS sufferer, the diabetic or the cancer patient, and do not present a united front. Indeed, the existence of patient advocates as well as advice and liaison groups indicate that their voices are weaker than they might be and requires advocacy to be heard in decision making.

In a similar way clinical staff groups differ and are often described as being in silos or tribes who protect their professional identity (such as nurses and doctors). This is also seen in occupational labels used, such as professions allied to medicine (note the implied centrality of the medical profession). This group includes physiotherapists, occupational therapists, speech therapists, plaster technicians, operating department assistants and dieticians. These too might stand apart from other ancillary staff groups, such as domestics, porters and catering teams, especially during pay and conditions negotiations, even though they all contribute to the success of the service.

The way in which internal groups express their roles suggests that a hierarchy exists between front-line and support-services stakeholders. Those not working at the staff – service user interface also contribute to the wider service operation, for example non-clinical managers, administrators, information managers, infection prevention staff, clinical governance teams, and audit and risk managers.

Residing over the internal stakeholders is the service executive team who might be answerable to a board of trustees. Their function sits at the interface between internal operations and formulating responses to external stakeholders, including the wider public (not necessarily just service user pressure groups), economists, politicians, professional groups and regulatory bodies.

Whilst the public, and particularly service users, should be key stakeholders the reality within complex health service delivery is that multiple competing voices shape what actually happens. Recognising this will help you to make decisions that acknowledge what can and cannot easily be changed. Furthermore, internal stakeholders need to be managed and is a function that often falls to local staff to maintain good inter-professional workplace relationships. At a higher level formal commissions exist to ensure that public stakeholder involvement is strengthened. I include an illustration from the Commission for Patient and Public Involvement in Health (CPPIH)[3] which was set up in January 2003 as an independent, non-departmental public body, sponsored by the Department of Health. The Commission's role is to make sure the public is involved in decision making about health and health services in England.

> These forums were subsequently abolished following public consultation as part of the Local Government and Public Involvement in Health Act 2007on 31 March 2008 and replaced by Local Involvement Networks (LINks).[4]

The aim of Local Involvement Networks is

> 'to give citizens a stronger voice in how their health and social care services are delivered. Run by local individuals and groups and independently supported – the role of LINks is to find out what people want, monitor local services and to use their powers to hold them to account.'[5]

Given that a statement needs to be made about 'citizen' stakeholder involvement, it suggests that the service can be owned and led by others, and LINks is an initiative to inform policy making, but it is not the only means of raising debate and challenging existing policy.

Perhaps now what you already hinted at in your letter is being affirmed in that service ownership is subject to stakeholder perspectives that shape service focus. As a manager you are located at the staff – service user interface within a series of contexts that are subject to change, some more and some less stable than others. This presents you with a challenge, but one that can be faced if you appreciate the big picture. Whilst decision making is complex, it is necessary to recognise the process followed to be able to demonstrate your rationale. Have a go at sketching out your decision-making process with respect to stakeholder involvement. This may be difficult because often decision making does not make the process used explicit, but doing this can clarify precisely who is involved and what their contribution is – in this way you might revisit your interpretation of whose service it is and its focus.

Yours truly,
Cartmel

Coffee break: decisions and stakeholders

You will be making service delivery decisions that are linked to each area of the organisation depicted in the model. These decisions will acknowledge stakeholder involvement and be bounded in certain ways.

- Revisit your description of the decision-making process in relation to stake-holder involvement. A diagram might help to clarify which steps are used in the process.

- What role and information might each identified stakeholder contribute to your decision making?

- How can you access the information that each stakeholder provides?

- What types of decisions do the stakeholders make? How might this be useful to know when making service delivery decisions?

LETTER 7: THE BIG PICTURE – WHAT IS THE MEANING OF HEALTH IN A HEALTH SERVICE?

Dear Marie,

Different factors shape your decision making apart from the process itself and stakeholder involvement. One of these is the meaning of health and it might be assumed that this is a stable definition that has universal agreement. I pose to you the question therefore: What is the meaning of health in a health service? Healthcare decision making is nothing new, indeed centuries ago Herodotus noted in his observations in Babylon:

> They have no doctors, but bring their invalids out on the street, where anyone who comes along offers the sufferer advice on his complaint, either from personal experience or observation of a similar complaint in others. Anyone will stop by the sick man's side and suggest remedies which he has himself proved successful in whatever the trouble may be, or which he has known to succeed in other people. Nobody is allowed to pass a sick person in silence, but everyone must ask him what is the matter.[1]

This illustration of decision making focuses on the 'invalid', who is at the mercy of chance (whoever might pass) and competing knowledge (their ideas and experience). At least there is an implied duty of care in so much as passers-by had to engage with the sick person. The invalid and not the passer decided (self-assessment) that a problem existed and that help was needed. This is a useful illustration if we are concerned about our own health and the health of others. We need to make some clear decisions about the meaning of health, and a means of recognising a health issue or deviation from a notion of health so it (ill health) can be labelled, in order to generate responses (evidence-based interventions) and recognise the obligations of a duty of care (so that a mandate is given to act).

Herodotus' writing also reveals a decision-making process – a decision-maker with a duty of care and understanding of health; decision stages including assessment, an intervention plan (based on evidence) and collaboration during implementation as the sick person had to choose to accept the advice or reject it. Further additions can be made to the process to explain what is assumed – all decisions draw upon and process information to generate decision options. Action on a chosen option will subsequently generate an outcome that in turn will provide further information for decision evaluation. We know that context influences each step, hence the decision-making model has real world value as the process represented in it encompasses the interplay of several elements rather than being purely linear.

Herodotus' account also raises questions about human experience in relation to health, the nature of people and their life experience. It prompts us to consider what enhances or detracts from their lived experience? What rights and needs do people have, and how can these be identified and understood? Is there a difference between want, need and right? Is there a social obligation to help others? If I am my brother's keeper what contribution can I make? How do we know that what we do actually helps others? These questions are relevant to our understanding of health and responsibility for health interventions.

It might be assumed that everyone can recognise what health is and is not, and so share a common understanding. However, a diverse range of views exist which I will briefly touch on.

To some the nature of a person – our nature – is a merely a physical machine that has evolved through successive generations to its current transitional state. This machine has the capacity for social and autonomous action. At death, however, it ceases to exist and returns to dust. This can sit comfortably with a biological, psychological and social model of health. Human existence is bounded between birth and death, and any interest in an individual's health lies within the span of these two events. But this secular view neglects the spiritual nature of person and the possibility of life being something far greater than a chance evolutionary event. Indeed, a perspective that accepts intelligent divine design and post death existence locates a finite lifespan within a coherent framework that explains the experience of people as spiritual, physical and social beings within a relationship to something beyond self, often called God. This is nothing new and in an ancient Hebrew book attributed to King Solomon entitled Ecclesiastes you will read of a study undertaken of 'everything that goes on under the sun'. In it Solomon generated a sequence of interim conclusions concerning the meaninglessness of life and concluded his argument stating that the temporal situation is only rendered meaningful when the vista is broadened out to include man's spiritual context in relation to God (recognising the nature of self), creation (recognising the context) and other people (the social world). It's up to you to study this further, but suffice to say that how we understand who and what we are will shape our world view, a framework of interpretation that we apply to understand the world around us and particularly health.

Health could be merely a physical matter of atoms, molecules, chemicals and systems that function in a predictable way. Ill health is diagnosed when a deviation is detected in relation to an 'atlas of the body' describing normal physical function. This is reminiscent of the medical model. Nurse recruits in the 1940s were subject to their health being classified in this way as noted in Ashdown's explanation of the qualities of a (healthy) nurse:[2]

> 'Good health and the absence of any of the following conditions are essential: Decayed teeth; offensive nasal discharge; otorrhoea; bromidrosis; or any other unhealthy taint.'

From here, it is only a short step to regarding physical health as a commodity. A body system can malfunction and an intervention (such as surgery) can restore this function. Healthcare provision associated with this perspective would support a purchaser-provider system that potentially raises barriers to care (on grounds of insufficient funds) or ease of access (provision being located in a geographically different area) or via arbitrary rules requiring some health behaviour being demonstrated before services are provided (such as losing weight, stopping tobacco or alcohol use). Both this and the previous view render it possible to locate health within the control of the individual and blame them if they become unhealthy.

Parsons[3] described health as a 'state of optimum capacity of an individual for the effective role and tasks for which he has been socialised'. An inability to function according to Parsons, would lead to the adoption of the sick role, which excused them from the expectation of functioning. Health as function lends itself to labeling and measurement.

When revisiting a holistic view of health there is room to consider spiritual aspects of health. Naturally, an understanding of the meaning of spirit is required (can it be alive or is it dead, strengthened or weakened?) as well as its relationship to decision making, hope and despair. This can be recognised in Plato's account of the trial and death of Socrates in which we read of a view of the existence of life beyond death to the extent that he faced his death sentence not with fear but anticipation. He eventually took his own life (with hemlock).

A distinction can be made between well-being and spiritual health. Well-being as a state of health describes a current experience and how one interprets it. This accent on experience is evident in press advertisements using words such as calming, relaxing and equilibrium. It also features in the 1946 World Health Organisation constitution that stated:[4]

> 'Health is a state of complete physical, mental and social well-being and not merely the absence of disease and infirmity.'

This leads us to a view of health as a positive state rather than merely what is left in the absence of deviation from an atlas of health. It follows that complete physical, mental and social well-being is an ideal state because any one deficit diminishes the whole. If there was always something that diminished any of these domains then it is possible that a person could always strive towards 'health', but may never attain it. In this case it seems that a state of incomplete health always exists. This raises some quite interesting problems, as defining 'completeness' in the three domains is contextually and culturally determined, therefore it is open to difference. This would render a definition of health unstable because there is the potential for multiple interpretations of the meaning of health. If health is a construct and not an absolute state it renders visionary documents such as 'Health for all' (WHO 2000)[5] problematic on account of it being actually less precise than their definition supposes. This has implications for the type of service required.

The excerpt from Herodotus served to illustrate factors shaping healthcare decision making. King Solomon provided a holistic context to understand human experience whilst Socrates gave an example of how an individual could make sense of their existence. These serve to aid our understanding of healthcare by recognising that different interpretations of health exist in decision making. Furthermore, the information deemed relevant to decision making will be informed by the dominant interpretation of health. So how do you understand the meaning of health?

Yours truly,
Cartmel

Coffee break: interpreting the meaning of health

There are different interpretations of health. Whichever is adopted will directly shape service purpose and design. It will also inform the design of measures to evaluate whether or not health interventions have been effective. So what is the dominant interpretation of health in your local service?

- Locate an explicit account of how the organisation expresses and therefore interprets the meaning of health.

- Do different interpretations exist within different parts of the organisation?

- If so, how do these find expression, and what are the implications for service design and delivery?

Decision maker at the heart of service delivery – you as manager?

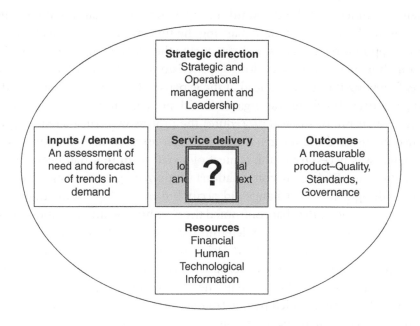

LETTER 1:   WHAT DO HEALTHCARE MANAGERS DO?

Dear Marie,

If a particular interpretation of health lies at the heart of health service design, then the work of a manager is also aligned to this. We can develop our understanding of what a manager does through reflection on experience. I will recount the example of a day surgery unit that historically admitted patients at 8 am for a full-day operating list of procedures conducted under either sedation or local anaesthetic. A hive of activity lasted for about an hour when all were seen and prepared for their procedure. This was often followed by a four-hour wait because the surgeon would typically commence his schedule with a 'major' operation on an inpatient. During this wait patients would be anxious, sometimes angry, and would give feedback about 'obvious' ways of improving how the service could be run. The surgeon's rationale for keeping a ward full of day patients waiting was 'just in case the major operation was cancelled'. The latter part of the day would involve another intensive period of activity when the ward was full of recovering patients awaiting discharge.

There was much that the day ward manager could do regarding the quality of service and workflow regulation, enhancing the time available to provide information and support for patients, as well as reducing the pressure on staff to work intensively for short periods between long gaps. Historically the ward sister had been passive, following the surgeon's lead at the expense of patient experience and staff working practices. The focus was organisational, not patient-centric: if patients were 'seen' (had their minor surgical procedure) the process was considered acceptable; the outcome justified the means. A new manager assessed the situation to decide what change was necessary in the context of a staff team that had been socialised into a status quo. Their early conversations cautioned against change: 'you won't change anything will you?'. Change did occur, but not without some mustering of allies and waging of battles that confronted the non-holistic interpretation of health and the stakeholder dominance in determining operational processes.

So what can we learn from this? Using the model as a guide, the manager reviewed the day-to-day processes to ensure provision of a safe environment of care (element 1). Next, they had to evaluate the resources required to deliver the service (element 4); these included people (management supervision and professional development), equipment (safe and fit-for-purpose equipment), budgetary constraints (efficiency savings had to be made) and information (for evidence-based practice and service development). Forward planning required information about trends in the changing nature of day surgery and identification of new skills that needed to be learnt (as different case load and treatments were being introduced) along with forecasts of demand (element 3). The service that had been inherited relied on high levels of interpersonal skill in patient care, but was weak in terms of professional record keeping. To facilitate outcome measurement (element 4), a prior step that involved designing and implementing a new record system and folio of service standards that corresponded to care process stages was needed. This effectively highlighted the need to establish a visible approach to quality whilst building on existing team strengths. Finally, plans for future service development needed to harmonise with the strategic plan (element 5). Beyond the immediate hospital-based operation there were other stakeholders to consider: volunteers, existing benefactors (who funded some new developments) and primary care staff (general practitioners, health visitors, social workers and community nurses) who provided ongoing services following discharge (the circle around the model represents the external contexts).

In brief, the manager's role has many facets. Some managers perform set functions according to their place in the organisation, the organisation's place in a development cycle and local needs. Some of these roles include:

- Process manager
- Project manager
- Change manager
- Strategic manger
- Trouble-shooter manager

Referring to element 1 of the model, the point of service delivery requires mangers capable of ensuring ensure smooth daily operation of the service. This is <u>process management</u> – each day requires delivery of the same high quality service and when required, interventions to restore this state.

When daily operations are enhanced by the introduction of a new process or system, such as an electronic record, <u>project managers</u> are employed. Their role is time-limited to oversee the planning and successful implementation of a discrete project. A popular UK standard for project management is Prince 2[1] which is worth reading through to complement your learning. It is useful to notice that the Prince 2 methodology stresses an organised and controlled approach which is far preferable – in any management activity - to lunging from crisis to crisis.

<u>Change management</u> is a constant in a modern health service and you will find some guidance (based on an educational setting but nonetheless useful) at the JISC Change Management Info Kit website.[2] A change management model comprised of three aspects is provided: people, processes and culture, along with a narrative aimed at assisting the reader in finding a suitable approach to becoming an effective and professional manager. A popular depiction of change comprises three steps: unfreezing, moving and refreezing. The latter stage is now thought to merge into a process of continual improvement. This process differs from a three stage transition management process (Endings, Neutral Zone, New Beginnings) and deals with the psychological reorientation that staff must go through as they come to terms with a change, thereby making the argument that transition rather than change itself is the issue that staff resist.

Stages of change management [3]

Unfreezing: Creating the motivation to change by disconfirmation of the present state, creation of survival anxiety, then creation of psychological safety to overcome learning anxiety.

Moving: Learning new concepts, new meanings, and new standards by imitation of, and identification with, role models, scanning for solutions and trial-and-error learning.

Refreezing: Internalising new concepts, meanings, and standards by incorporating these into self-concept and identity as well as into ongoing relationships and groups.

Strategic management is allied to medium- and long-term change management in which key steps in managing the organisation's capabilities are to:[4]
- define business strategies and goals
- determine the competences needed to achieve those goals
- identify core competences (those competences that the organisation must have in-house)
- analyse current competences and identify gaps
- decide on sourcing strategy for addressing the gaps; options include bringing in new skills and improving competences of current staff
- monitor and manage ongoing requirements for organisational capability.

The strategic element of the whole operation will always need an executive eye casting over it to ensure that the integrated service complexity continues to align to the business plan. This executive's role is to monitor and intervene as necessary to ensure that agreed targets and contracts are met.

The trouble shooter manager takes an analytical approach to short assignments and is sent to 'sort out' a service for a few weeks or months. This person identifies issues and devises action plans to resolve them. You might observe this role in action in service delivery in health and education sectors when external managers are appointed to directly manage or support an existing management team to bring a failing service back to a required standard.

So, Marie, a short reflection can help us to recognise a manager's different roles according to the situation. Chiefly, managers have a responsibility to ensure that planned provision maintains a service user focus. This, of course, is different to management style which emphasises how you approach the role of being a manager. It is worth remembering that as an organisation moves through different development cycles different management roles will be 'front stage' and others 'back stage'.

Sometimes organisations undergo restructuring which can entail closing some services, retraining and redeploying staff and opening new services. Such times of turbulence require skilled change management for a season. Once the changes have been achieved and are embedded, a different management style is needed as stability and consolidation become the order of the day and process managers reoccupy a 'front stage' role.

It follows that whatever the front stage role of the moment there are associated decisions which fall into two categories corresponding to the model provided:

- Decisions about maintaining service operation (ensuring that agreed processes are effectively and efficiently followed each day).
- Decisions about changing service operation (altering work processes to adapt to the changing patterns of demand or changing what is needed in different elements of the model).

Marie, your decision making as a manager is informed by determining whether your role is concerned with continuity or change, and the relative balance between the two. So what do you do as a manager and what is your principal role?

Kind regards

Cartmel

Coffee break: what are your management roles and competencies?

This extended reflection leads you to consider the range of management roles and where your emphasis currently lies. Then you are asked to consider how a folio of competencies relates to your various roles. Whilst the Key Skills framework is cited as an example it is not the only competency framework possible, nor is it necessarily comprehensive enough to meet all of your development needs. Indeed, your development is likely to be broader than a limited organisational focus on staff fulfilling their role descriptions.

> What are your management roles?
>
> What do you think are your major and minor management roles? Identify these roles in relation to each element of the model.

Which management role competencies do you need?

Next read about the Key Skills Framework to identify some competencies linked to the roles that you have identified. This framework is described as a 'single, consistent, comprehensive and explicit framework on which to base review and development

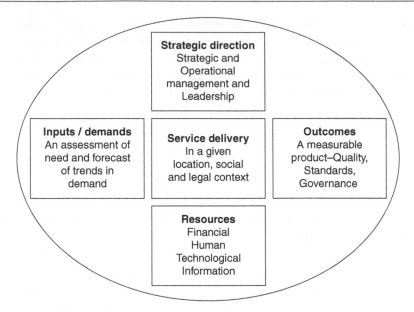

FIGURE 6 The model used to identify roles

for all staff.'[1] It has six core and four specific dimensions. The six core dimensions can be linked to sections of the model, although more competencies exist than are identified within the KSF.

Here is how I think that this maps onto the model. All elements of a healthcare organisation require effective communication within and across the model (integrated 5 element model – dimension 1), services are delivered through a well trained workforce (element 5 resources – dimension 2) and are provided safely in a risk managed environment (element 5 resources, element 1 service delivery – dimension 3); there is a continuous quality cycle of development (outcomes elements 1, 4 and 5 – dimension 4) that is measurable (element 4 – dimension 5) and respects the legal rights of participants (element 1 – dimension 6). The KSF competencies are given for your reference:[2]

Core dimensions
Six dimensions are core to the working of every NHS job:
1 Communication
2 Personal and people development
3 Health, safety and security
4 Service development
5 Quality
6 Equality, diversity and rights.

Specific dimensions
There are a further 24 specific dimensions which can be applied to define parts of different posts. These are grouped into four categories:

1   Health and well-being (HWB 1–10)
2   Information and knowledge (IK 1–3)
3   General (G 1–8)
4   Estates and facilities (EF 1–3).

You might find it useful to read the RCN guidance for nurses and managers in creating KSF outlines in the NHS.[3]

How big is the task?

The following summary (from the NHS graduate scheme) illustrates the magnitude of the manager's task. Read this in the context of the model provided to see where the narrative corresponds to its elements and consider what is 'best management' and which competency set would match this.

> As the biggest single organisation in Europe, the NHS employs 1.3 million people and has an annual budget of around £90 billion. Within it there are hundreds of organisations – Primary Care Trusts, Acute Trusts, Foundation Trusts, Mental Health Trusts and others - each with their own management boards and budgets. And good management directly affects patient care.
>
> Set up on the 5th July 1948, the National Health Service – the NHS – has experienced huge changes to both its organisational structure and the way that patient services are provided. But despite ever-increasing pressures, to this day it remains true to its founding principle of providing healthcare for all based on need, not the ability to pay.
>
> A 24/7, 365 days a year operation, the NHS is the second largest Government spending programme. Think of its sheer size this way; if the NHS was a country, it would be 33rd in the OECD list of countries with the biggest economies! The NHS is implementing state-of-the-art management processes, systems and techniques to give patients more choice and better information, underpinned by new financial systems, all requiring effective management. At the same time, systems to support clinical staff need improving so that their pressured time is used most effectively.
>
> Investment in healthcare since 1997 will have trebled by 2008. We are a growing business. We are also radically changing the way we work to offer patients much more choice about how they receive care. We will be bringing more care closer to home and using new technology and innovations to raise quality and improve productivity. Our reform programme is far-reaching and complex.

> Meeting this massively complex challenge calls for the best management and leadership on the market today and in the future.
>
> NHS Graduate Scheme[4]

By the end of this extended reflection you will have identified your roles and role competencies, and considered the scope of the management task.

LETTER 2: HOW DO MANAGERS MANAGE?

Dear Marie,

If a manager has a number of different roles that vary according to the requirements of the situation, then the way in which the manager undertakes those roles is at the heart of facilitating management in practice. I have come across a number of managers who operate under a cloak of mystique – their practice is to have all of their management knowledge 'in their head' and disclose very little. In such cases the acquisition of knowledge becomes a threat as it renders a previously unassailable position vulnerable by opening up the possibility of someone else being able to perform the manager's function.

Consider the newly qualified staff member who is attempting to map out a personal development pathway. They need to know what it is that they should know to advance their portfolio of experience in order to mature professionally. The manager who keeps knowledge locked up 'in their head' is unlikely to disclose much at all to facilitate such a pathway and this is where a model can be beneficial. It offers a means of mapping domains where knowledge needs to be gained so that the new staff member knows where to begin their enquiries.

Take, for example resource management; the whole trajectory of developing role specifications, role costing, recruitment, induction, retention and staff development, and eventually of overseeing those leaving employment requires specific knowledge. Mapping this trajectory will provide you with reference points from which to seek out additional information and corresponding experience. Let's select recruitment and the interview process as one point on the trajectory. You will need to be aware of how to plan an interview, establish how the panel will conduct it, arrange the venue and individual candidate schedule and assess candidates in a fair and transparent way. Equally, you will need to know what is not legally permissible to ask (equal opportunities), make a decision, inform candidates of the outcome and make an offer of appointment subject to conditions.

When you map out the recruitment and interview process in this level of detail you will be facilitating your own development because you will learn (or remind yourself) what it is you need to ask, read or access training about. In this way you could create your own development list in a professional portfolio so that each working experience can be seen as an opportunity to gain new insights.

Now, let's return to my point about the manager who retains management knowledge mystique by avoiding information disclosure. You will be aware that gaining such knowledge could be perceived as a threat and that some managers are threatened to the extent that they withhold information from others. The saying, 'knowledge is power' is illustrated in the type of manager who strengthens their own position by surrounding themselves with a group comprising those 'in the know' who in turn act as information gatekeepers. You will have heard the term 'being kept out of the loop' to describe this scenario. I heard an experienced manager once advise, upon reflection, to choose a manager carefully. That placed a different emphasis on an interview and introduced the notion of it being a two-way assessment – the candidate might evaluate the interview experience as indicative of an organisation that is not right for them. This prompts questions about management styles and to answer these we need to focus on the heart of the role – the nature of people.

If we can understand what we are like, then we can anticipate how we might act and react in given situations; this will directly shape how we actually manage. I will close with an illustration from military service of what really matters in managing (and leading) others. Following months of training and acquisition of technical knowledge, Royal Navy officer recruits were mustered in a lecture theatre. The career ahead was outlined, with its challenges, excitement and potential dangers. The idea of success focused on what really gets results; a sailor marched onto the stage and stood facing the assembled company. 'This gentlemen, is the most important factor – the sailor who serves with you.' Understanding people and your approach to them is a key to answering the question: How do managers manage? So also for you Marie, at the heart of management, are those who serve with you. Care for them and your experience will be altogether richer.

Yours truly,
Cartmel

Coffee break: understanding people to manage people

The skill of understanding human nature and reading behaviour lies at the heart of management. It is not enough to be a manager who is technically excellent regarding systems and process; a manager with a portfolio of task-specific abilities but who lacks essential 'people skills' will be less effective than one who understands their co-workers and staff. This reflection is really an ongoing issue to keep revisiting. It is about the immensely absorbing appreciation of people and learning how to work with them, and around them.

- Which information sources do you access to learn about people, their nature and their behaviour?
- What is the nature of a person?
- What do you base your perspective on?
- How sufficient is this perspective?

- What is the implication of your perspective in terms of translating it into actions based on truthfulness, collaboration, fairness, transparency, advocacy, firmness?

- How do you manage situations where there exists a diversity of perspectives about the nature of a person?

LETTER 3: HIT THE GROUND RUNNING?

Dear Marie,

If we understand what a manger does and how they approach managing people then we have the recipe for effective management. So can you really just move into a new post and 'hit the ground running'? This term is current management speak that means to undertake a role on arrival in a new post without any need for extensive induction or additional training and development. It sounds like the ideal, cost-effective appointment to a post: just arrive and do the job that is required.

As a manager you need to ask: In which situations would this actually apply? And what knowledge, skills and experience is required for the appointee to achieve this starting point? Having reflected on this, is it possible to actually 'hit the ground running'?

I think not. All organisations are different and employ different methods and processes, possess individual cultures or mindsets, and have a range of personalities. If you need to work with people then it is important to 'walk' with those people to find out about them. In the armed services, officer recruits are given a cook's tour of every department to allow them to gain insight into the work and perspectives of others; new commanding officers still have to orient themselves to their crews. Therefore, managing is more than having excellent organisational skills, and leadership is more than giving orders. It is the same in a healthcare service context – a new staff member will still need to appreciate the context in which they are working and that is learned through experience as much as through oral briefings.

I suggest that you recognise your skills and market them in a confident manner so that when used in practice (some might refer to this as 'hitting the ground running'), you proceed purposefully. Sensitivity to a new context will add to your appreciation of its nuances. This will contribute to the way in which you undertake your work as a manager and you might walk more confidently, even appearing to proceed more briskly at a measured pace. This is different to the stop-start rush of enthusiasm that runs ahead of clear thinking about your work. So are you or your employees able to hit the ground running?

Yours truly,
Cartmel

Coffee break: role continuity or change?

If you had a skills deficit in a team you could employ the right person to fit the requirement – the round peg for the round hole. That is useful and can happen in cases where short term relief cover is required (such as a six-month maternity leave). Consider what additional value might be gained through the practice of managing others by accepting that a post is more than 'a peg in a hole'; recognise that the 'hole' might need to be refashioned and the 'peg' altered to match the new requirement.

- Can you detect any assumptions about how the local organisation under-stands the role of the manager?
- What indications are there that this is up for negotiation by post holders?
- What is the process by which this might be achieved?
- How would a change in the manager's role impact on other aspects of the model?
- In cases where the scope of the manager's role is not negotiable, what is the organisation likely to lose and gain?

LETTER 4: DECISION MAKING AND CHANGE – READING THE ENVIRONMENT

Dear Marie,

We won't be hitting any ground running at the moment. Autumn has turned into winter and it is snowing, the pavements have a crisp white mantle and drifts are collecting in doorways and against the parapets of the nearby canal bridge. There is change in the air and office workers have begun to leave work early before public transport is disrupted.

We can read the signs around us to anticipate change. When I went to the main post office this morning there was a chill easterly wind. Across the skyline was a bank of grey-laden clouds and I knew that shortly they would begin to dump their snow across the city. Within half an hour light snow flurries had arrived, heralding a short lived blizzard. This reminded me of the time when I was part of a military expedition team on the ascent of Galdhoppigen, one of Norway's higher peaks (at 2469 metres) in the Jotunheim range, the 'home of the Giants.' A blizzard swept in just as we neared the summit. There was nothing that we could do to avoid it, save hope to reach a stone booth before it struck. We didn't, and being caught out in the open, we experienced a whiteout, which is a situation of zero visibility in all directions.

So why am I writing to you about snow in the city and being at the top of a Norwegian mountain when you are in a cosy ward in a centrally-heated urban hospital? Well, when a sudden crisis causes you to temporarily lose all reference points, your decision making strategy has to take over so that you can formulate a safe, purposeful plan of action that draws on a range of information sources to produce a required outcome.

A situation analysis facilitated recognition of decision options. We were on a mountain snow field in the proximity of a cornice (a wind-blown snow overhang) that we were in danger of falling through should we venture onto it. We were unlikely to survive falling off the edge of a mountain in blizzard conditions, especially as we were an independent team a few days' trek away from base camp.

When in the midst of a complex situation with multiple dimensions, it is possible to feel overwhelmed by a sudden storm that sweeps in. But that does not mean that your thinking has to be paralysed or your knowledge cast aside. Granted, there are situations so unexpected that your thinking can be momentarily numbed, but hopefully your training will kick in and you will take charge and make decisions rather than allow events to make them for you.

Whilst 'time and chance happen to all people'[1] and sweeps in under various guises, such as war, epidemic or economic collapse, changes can be detected as they approach and it is good to be able to read both the internal clinical landscape (within your organisation) and the external environment (policy, economic, social changes and trends) to anticipate their likely impact. We all need to be adept at reading the internal and external environments to identify change.

So what steps can you take?

- Read the external and internal environments – Question trends and antici-pate what their impact will be. In the case of the blizzard, we knew it was approaching and that it could leave us stranded on the mountain. We had a mental checklist: What did we know about our current situation? What were our position, rations, equipment? How many hours of daylight were left? Where could we create a shelter? Checking the facts of what you know will clarify the current position by determining what has changed (in the bliz-zard example, the weather; in a healthcare organization, perhaps a major disaster that poses a clear threat to service continuity).
- Assess the impact this change will have – A prolonged blizzard on a moun-tain might necessitate sheltering until it abates – possibly a night in a snow hole. But a delay will impact on other resources such as rations and cook-ing fuel.
- Generate options and select one to act upon – Recognise the options you have. We agreed on an immediate short-term plan (shelter and wait for the storm to pass), and a medium-term plan (prepare an overnight shelter if dusk had fallen before the blizzard abated and make the descent when the weather cleared the next day). The choice between the two options was dependent upon the duration of the blizzard.
- Act – Implement agreed decisions and evaluate progress.

Reflection on previous experience can add to your learning and hone your ability to read the external environment to evaluate the implications for change in the inter-nal environment. You could also ask which signs that were evident in retrospect were not initially recognised as indicators of change, and how this shaped your decision options. What alternative courses of action could have been taken, and did any actions cause more problems than solutions?

Well, Marie, you will probably have a major incident plan at work based on an analysis of anticipated threats to service continuity. This indicates that thought has already gone into reading what might happen in the external service deliv-ery environment and how the internal service environment should respond in an organised way. During your coffee break examine that plan. I'm going to post this before the snow brings the city to a standstill and local services implement their major incident plans.

Yours,
Cartmel

Coffee break: reading the environment

Use this break to do two tasks:

1   Identify current changes in the external environment (use a PEST framework

Political, Economic, Social, Technological dimensions) and use the guide below to think through what the implications for local actions might be.

Use this guide –

(a) Read the external and internal environments

(b) Assess the impact of the trends and indicators you identify that need to be addressed

(c) Generate options

(d) Act

Then look through your local major incident plan to see the scope of events included and the procedure for responding to it.

2 To add to the scope of your knowledge about major incident planning check out relevant on-line guidance beginning with the resources offered below. You will find more examples of healthcare disaster plans in the public domain.
   a. Planning for the evacuation and sheltering of people in health sector settings: interim strategic national guidance[1]
   b. Examples of good practice in emergency planning[2]
   c. You might consider how process safety thinking can provide a robust approach to planning – The Health and Safety Executive has advice publicly available.[3]

Decision making at the point of service delivery

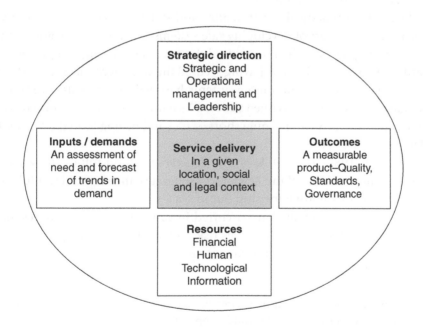

LETTER 1:   MANAGING PROCESSES – GOVERNANCE

Dear Marie,

It might seem to some a bit of a chore undertaking local service audit checks, but I am reminded of how some local managers responded to an external inspection report. The inspector highlighted a lack of evidence to support the service's answers to questions about specific care processes, such as criminal records bureau checks on new staff and verification of their current professional registration status. It was that lack of awareness about the need for specific processes to be in place rather than the absence of actual records that raised concerns. This could be likened to local managers flying an aeroplane without having full control. A lack of attention to detail has predictable consequences, and a lack of process control will eventually harm staff, patients and public confidence in the service. Furthermore, neglect of care processes and systems effectively condones increased risk – hence what might seem like a chore is actually an essential frontline action that allows managers to identify and intervene appropriately to ensure operational compliance with systems-related policies and procedures.

We know that thinking about structures and systems does not excite everyone, but it is necessary as part of developing safe systems. After all, you would not want to fly on an aeroplane that had not passed the necessary pre-flight engineer checks or board a ferry without the crew having secured the watertight integrity of the ship. But people have done so, and unsafe systems have led to incidents. In September 2001 a transatlantic airline was fined $250 000 for improper maintenance work that resulted in the Airbus A 330 running short of fuel and having to make an unscheduled landing in the Azores.[1]

On 6 March 1987, *The Herald of Free Enterprise* roll-on-roll-off ferry took on board water and capsized off the Belgian coast because the crew did not fully close the bow doors before putting the ship out to sea.[2]

In a similar way, incidents have occurred in care settings that have resulted in a patient's death. One example involves risk assessment and management of beds and bed rails linked to patient entrapment and suffocation. This excerpt illustrates a cluster of such events:

> … the child became entrapped in an area between the mattress on the bed and the attached bed rail, in one case the child slipped through the bars of the bedrail, in another a child was found hanging from a protrusion on the bedrail itself, and 2 children were entrapped in the space between the headboard/bedpost and the bed rail. The deaths were the result of asphyxia or strangulation…[3]

Cases where an accidental death verdict was pronounced, as when an 'Elderly patient died on trolley in understaffed hospital'[4] highlight resource issues associated with maintaining safe systems of care. These illustrations emphasise the need for the design and management of safe systems, and no less so where patient care is concerned. For care managers, patient care and systems care are mutually inter-twined, – they are not binary choices. So where do we need to focus our thoughts when examining frontline service management?

A logical starting point from the point of view of your role in service delivery is to appreciate the big picture of service organisation (as provided in the model that we are familiar with), so that any local system development can be understood in relation to it. The central element of the systems model represents the integration of managing the care environment, the organisation of care delivery and the team who deliver care. I will consider these aspects in turn.

Managing the environment of care

Descriptions of what constitutes a care environment – regardless of whether it is a ward, a community clinic, a vehicle, or a person's home – are valuable in appreciating the specific tasks included in its management. Knowledge of these is nothing new; indeed, back in 1880 Florence Nightingale explained aspects of this in her *Notes on Nursing*.[5] Tasks were associated with ensuring the provision of pure air, water, efficient drainage, cleanliness and light. The essence of her notes have a contemporary resonance owing to her explanation of the need for some-one to manage the patient's care environment (the tasks being regulating heating, light, noise, waste disposal and hygiene). That translates into the modern era as hotel services management, and infection prevention and control. Furthermore, Florence Nightingale also explained how the patient required management of their social context of care – social interaction, interruptions to daily routines, diet, exercise, observation and the extent of their participation in care. This trans-lates into contemporary practice as managing a bespoke care plan or pathway to guide and monitor the patient's progression along a set trajectory. Recalling how I commenced this letter by commenting on audit and inspection, external regula-tory requirements exist to ensure that providers have specific processes in place to ensure patient safety. These have a legal basis and are approved in the United Kingdom by Parliament. Compliance is checked through an audit process. Each provider should have an internal audit function that oversees compliance check-ing and generates reports that are useful in identifying good practice, and to target interventions in non-compliant areas to ensure standards are met. Care manage-ment also includes external inspection. In the United Kingdom the Care Quality Commission was established by the Health and Social Care Act 2008 to regulate the quality of health and social care, and to look after the interest of people detained under the Mental Health Act.[6]

> From April 2009, the Care Quality Commission has responsibility for registering, reviewing and inspecting services. Its aim is to 'help services improve by ensuring standards are met and that bad practice is stamped out and do this is by using our enforcement powers.' Where providers of services fail to meet the legal requirements of their registration action may be taken against them.

The CQC powers include issuing warning notices, impose, vary or remove conditions, issue a penalty notice in lieu of prosecution, suspend registration, cancel registration and prosecute for specified offences.

External inspection can result in fines being levied for certain offences. These include failure to be registered (incurs a £50 000 fine), obstructing an inspector, failure to provide documents or information, and failure to provide an explanation of any related matter (each incurs a fine of £2 500).[7]

We can see that this is to be taken seriously and the regulator's requirements need to be translated into auditable practice. To help this process, reference is made to guidance and codes. Health legislation guidance is usually provided to aid interpretation of the law and statutory requirements. Whilst it is not mandatory, if followed it would normally help organisations to do enough to comply with the law. Approved Codes of Practice offer practical examples of good practice and advice on how to comply with the law, with guides to what is 'reasonably practicable' and illustrations of how this can apply in specific circumstances.

The Health and Safety Executive (HSE) advises that Approved Codes of Practice 'have a special legal status. If employers are prosecuted for a breach of health and safety law, and it is proved that they have not followed the relevant provisions of the Approved Code of Practice, a court can find them at fault unless they can show that they have complied with the law in some other way'.[8]

Therefore, managing the care environment necessitates identifying the relevant Acts of Parliament (or equivalent when working in other countries), codes and guidance, and then mapping where existing processes address these. It follows that governing the care environment requires detailed knowledge of these processes. Health and Safety regulations need to be consulted together with the support of designated health and safety staff within your organisation to understand the specifics about what you must do. Primary resources can be found at the Health and Safety Executive web pages[9] on which you can read about the relationship between Acts and Statutory Instruments.

The primary legislation comprises the Acts of Parliament, including the Health and Safety at Work Act 1974. The secondary legislation is made up of Statutory Instruments (SIs), often referred to as 'regulations'. It is enforced by HSE and Local Authorities (LAs). HSE and LAs work locally, regionally and nationally to common objectives and standards.

Let's take a practical example to show how legislation translates into safe practice. The Control of Substances Hazardous to Health Regulation (2002) (COSHH)[10] information pages provide guidance on how to comply with this regulation.

A web-based resource, 'COSHH Essentials, has been developed to help firms comply with the Control of Substances Hazardous to Health Regulations (COSHH)'. It goes on to advise that COSHH requires employers to:

- assess the risks to health from chemicals and decide what controls are needed
- use those controls and make sure workers use them
- make sure the controls are working properly
- inform workers about the risks to their health; train workers.

Other hazards present themselves in everyday practice because not everything is approached in a methodical way (although it is advantageous to do so), and it is worth reflecting on how workplace familiarity can be associated with failing to recognise risks. You will see evidence of this where fire equipment is covered by furniture or rubbish sacks, fire doors are wedged open, hazardous substances are not stored in an appropriate secure area and personal protective clothing, although provided, is not used. I once visited a South Yorkshire coal mine to observe colliers' working conditions and noted how ear defenders were not used because they were considered to be an inconvenience – perhaps you have seen road workers doing the same. This, however, represents the provision of personal protective equipment and 'employees have legal responsibilities to cooperate with their employer's efforts to improve health and safety'. Another example involving taking high-risk shortcuts involved some coal miners who, instead of walking along a roadway away from the coal face to a mine shaft, would risk riding on a coal conveyor belt (strictly forbidden), and as a consequence an incident did occur in which a miner had his arm severed off.

At this point it is worth mentioning risk assessment and what it entails. Please take time to read the resources about risk management available on the HSE website.[11] There are five steps to undertaking a risk assessment. These are:

1 identify the hazards
2 decide who might be harmed and how
3 evaluate the risks and decide on precautions
4 record your findings and implement them
5 review your assessment and update if necessary.

When thinking about your risk assessment, remember: 'a *hazard* is anything that may cause harm, such as chemicals, electricity, working from ladders, an open drawer etc.; the *risk* is the chance, high or low, that somebody could be harmed by these and other hazards, together with an indication of how serious the harm could be'.[12]

So how does this work out in practice? I will illustrate this by recalling a story where a new outpatient department manager noticed that a liquid nitrogen flask was stored in a patient examination room. This insulated metal flask had a cork bung and was routinely handled by staff to decant some of the contents into a dish for use in a skin treatment clinic. This practice was an accepted feature of work in the outpatient department that was not questioned. When examined with 'fresh eyes' hazards were identified that included a lack of protection against a substance that was clearly harmful to health, its method of storage in an unsecured (non-compliant) flask, its storage in a room with public access and without appropriate ventilation. The risks were that when handling the flask or knocking it over a person could be injured owing to spillage of its contents and inhalation of its fumes. Potential risks included a member of the public knocking the flask over; children, who also used the examination room, could also have been injured, as the flask was stored on the floor under an examination couch.

The risks were all evaluated as high – there was a real chance that such accidents could actually happen. These findings of the assessment were recorded as part of the case to secure funding to ensure necessary changes were implemented.

The precautions that were devised and implemented included (i) providing an appropriate secure access, safe place of storage with a ventilation/extraction system; (ii) provision of a new screw-top flask housed in a handling frame; (iii) provision of personal protective equipment for staff (gloves, apron and face visor); (iv) provision of staff training to ensure they understood the safe handling and storage of this product. Once implemented, the Control of Substances Hazardous to Health (COSHH) review became part of that department's regular audit cycle.

Well, Marie, process management is not complicated; it is simply the application of a thoughtful approach to identifying risks and taking practical steps to reduce or remove them. Governance is a term applying to an integrated view of process and people management. During your coffee break I suggest that you examine more aspects of risk management and associated reporting.

Yours,
Cartmel

Coffee break: managing processes—governance and risk reporting

- Risk

As mentioned in the letter, it is relatively easy to work out which systems of care delivery are needed by referring to the relevant legislation and regulatory requirements. I have reproduced a summary of regulations relevant to the workplace provided by the HSE (2008). Employers are required to carry out risk assessments, make arrangements to implement necessary measures and appoint competent people as well as to arrange for appropriate information and training.

Select one of example from these regulations and examine the detail of what is included so that you can:

- understand how risk assessment related to these are undertaken in your workplace
- identify the measures to address the risks

- identify what training and information is provided in relation to those measures

- finally, consider how this regulation has been applied to yourself during your employment

A summary of regulations relevant to the workplace (HSE, 2008)[1]

1 *Management of Health and Safety at Work Regulations 1999:* require employers to carry out risk assessments, make arrangements to implement necessary measures, appoint competent people and arrange for appropriate information and training.

2 *Workplace (Health, Safety and Welfare) Regulations 1992:* cover a wide range of basic health, safety and welfare issues such as ventilation, heating, lighting, workstations, seating and welfare facilities.

3 *Health and Safety (Display Screen Equipment) Regulations 1992:* set out requirements for work with Visual Display Units (VDUs).

4 *Personal Protective Equipment at Work Regulations 1992:* require employers to provide appropriate protective clothing and equipment for their employees.

5 *Provision and Use of Work Equipment Regulations 1998:* require that equipment provided for use at work, including machinery, is safe.

6 *Manual Handling Operations Regulations 1992:* cover the moving of objects by hand or bodily force.

7 *Health and Safety (First Aid) Regulations 1981:* cover requirements for first aid.

8 *The Health and Safety Information for Employees Regulations 1989:* require employers to display a poster telling employees what they need to know about health and safety.

9 *Employers' Liability (Compulsory Insurance) Act 1969:* require employers to take out insurance against accidents and ill health to their employees.

10 *Reporting of Injuries, Diseases and Dangerous Occurrences Regulations 1995 (RID-DOR):* require employers to notify certain occupational injuries, diseases and dangerous events.

11 *Noise at Work Regulations 1989:* require employers to take action to protect employees from hearing damage.

12 *Electricity at Work Regulations 1989:* require people in control of electrical systems to ensure they are safe to use and maintained in a safe condition.

13 *Control of Substances Hazardous to Health Regulations 2002 (COSHH):* require employers to assess the risks from hazardous substances and take appropriate precautions.

- Reporting of injuries, diseases and dangerous occurrences regulations
  Certain accidents and diseases have to be reported under the Reporting of Injuries, Diseases and Dangerous Occurrences Regulations (1995). 'Reporting accidents and ill health at work is a legal requirement. The information enables

the Health and Safety Executive (HSE) and Local Authorities, to identify where and how risks arise, and to investigate serious accidents'.[1]

Look through the RIDDOR web pages (or equivalent if you are working in a different country) to know the criteria for making a report and how you would do this. These include deaths, major injuries, specific minor injuries and dangerous occurrences (near misses). For specific details see the web page.[2]

- Health and safety

The Health and Safety at Work Act 1974[3] explicitly outlines employer and employee responsibilities in the workplace. Ownership by staff of these responsibilities will happen when they understand safe working practices and how these can become part of everyday practice, hence the need for training. Look at the Heath and Safety Executive website to review the Act which is primary legislation, and secondary Acts called Statutory Instruments. I want you to specifically read the enforcement section within the website and look through examples of the three following types of enforcement – prosecutions, improvement notices and prohibition notices so that you gain an appreciation of what can happen and the fines imposed if this aspect of providing a safe working environment is neglected.

LETTER 2: GOVERNANCE AND SMART WORKING PROCESSES

Dear Marie,

Thanks for your feedback about some of the issues that hitherto had not been recognised but which you now realise are a part of the matrix of a safe care environment. Next I will turn your attention to how we can examine work processes with a view to improving efficiency and effectiveness. The primary care process is that of the patient travelling on their 'journey' through your service. By mapping out this journey you can identify each step, what happens, who is involved and which resources are used. Previous measures aimed at generating a seamless journey for the patient have included arranging the service configuration around this journey. Care pathways were also developed for specific types of patient to identify planned activities at each stage of the journey and who was involved.

Having a mere pathway alone doesn't automatically improve patient outcomes, although it will contribute to a coherent and integrated service. Care bundles, a more recent development from the US, is a structured method for improving care processes and patient outcomes, and is gradually being adopted in the UK. It involves a small set of practices (generally three to five) 'that, when performed collectively, reliably and continuously, have been proven to improve patient outcomes'.[1] The purpose, as explained by the Institute of Healthcare Improvement (IHI), is to 'make a process more reliable… by improving habits and processes' adding that 'a bundle is a specific tool with clear parameters'. This differs from some other audit processes by emphasising the importance of completing all important elements of care, rather than considering each individually. In this way clinical teams systematically examine their processes of care and focus on how therapeutic interventions are delivered rather than on the interventions themselves.[2]

Bundles and pathways are relevant, but I want to focus on the centrality of the patient's journey through the service. I will illustrate this with an example from a day case surgery service. The journey starts when a patient is seen in a community health centre by a general practitioner who decides whether or not a referral to a specialist is required. Let's assume that this is made to a particular specialist surgeon. The patient attends an appointment with the surgeon and following consultation the patient is offered a treatment and a place on a waiting list. A choose and book service is accessed to select a specific date for the operation and preparatory information is provided for the patient. On the specified date transport services (if required) collect the patient and convey them to the surgical centre. On arrival, the patient undergoes an admission assessment, and following the pre-operation preparations (perhaps medication, specific skin preparation and a medical staff visit to obtain written consent and conduct anaesthetic assessment) they wait for their turn on the operating schedule. The next step is a staff check at theatre reception, transfer into the theatre, anaesthetic room care, the operation, transfer into a recovery suite and subsequent return to the ward. Health monitoring takes place until such time that the patient is assessed as being fit to be discharged. Post-operation advice and a surgeon's report are provided, and transport arranged to take the patient home. Follow-up care is arranged and subsequent appointments made if required.

This process can be represented as a straight line, and around which participants' actions and resources can be identified. Mapping this facilitates asking questions – what? when? who? how? about the patient, process, participants and resources. The first three are descriptive while the fourth is more of a critique.

'What? when? and who?' questions include:

- Patients – Who are the patients? What is the patient's experience of this journey?
- Process – What is this process? When do delays occur? What delays occur at different points in the process? What causes these delays?
- Participants – Who are the participants and what is their involvement in this process?
- Resources – What resources are critical to the progression of this journey?

'How?' questions include:

- Patients – How do patients engage in this process?
- Process – How does the process work?
- Participants – How do the participants collaborate to enhance progress or encounter resistance that impede the patient journey?
- Resources – How are resources managed in order to support this process?

The outcome of mapping the patient journey and asking these types of questions is to identify emerging issues, such as points of delay, duplication of activity and information seeking from patients, so that purposeful interventions can be proposed and implemented to make the service relevant and robust in design around the patient. Such measures elevate the role of the manager (a person who operates existing processes efficiently and effectively) into a leadership role (where they alter the process or replace it with something different).

Associated with the patient journey are subprocesses concerning ways of working amongst staff groups. These too can be examined to assess how effective and efficient they are. Thus, whilst the grand narrative of the patient journey is a large undertaking, at a local level there are still processes that small groups of staff can examine and develop. One method is called lean thinking, which is an approach developed by a motor manufacturer (Toyota) to improve flow and eliminate waste. It is about getting the right things to the right place, at the right time and in the right quantities while minimising waste, and being flexible and open to change. 'Lean brings into many industries, including healthcare, new concepts, tools and methods that have been effectively utilised to improve process flow. Tools that address workplace organisation, standardisation, visual control and elimination of non-value added steps are applied to improve flow, eliminate waste and exceed customer expectations'.[4] Lean thinking has five principles to enhance the quality of healthcare by improving flow in the patient journey and eliminating waste. These are[5]

1   Specify value – Value is any activity which improves the patient's health, well-being and experience. This might be less waiting and delay, better outcomes or fewer adverse incidents.
2   Identify the patient journey – The set of actions required to deliver value for patients.
3   Make the process and value flow – This means aligning healthcare processes to facilitate a smooth 'flow' of patients along the care pathway and also information.
4   Let the customer pull – This means that every step in the patient journey needs to pull people, skills, materials and information towards it as required. This implies that care delivery should be demand driven along with the resources needed for it.
5   Pursue perfection – This means that there should be a continuous process of evaluation and review to develop processes in pursuit of the ideal.

The terminology chosen seems somewhat commercial in its tone and could be 'interpreted' for a healthcare setting as (i) deciding what a good service would look like; (ii) identify the patient journey; (iii) rearrange the service around that journey; (iv) make patient need the determining factor on how the service should be configured at any given stage; (v) finally, continue to seek improvements. Lean thinking focuses on reducing identified types of waste in work processes. These are: correction (of faulty processes and repetition), waiting (stages where people are unable to process their work), transportation (when materials are moved unnecessarily), overprocessing (where there are unnecessary process steps), inventory (too much work in progress), motion (too much movement due to things not being accessible) and overproduction (producing more than is needed by the next process).

By adopting a process approach you can make real inroads into the efficiency of your service. Another practical approach allied to this is called 'The Productive Ward', which is a practical work programme aimed at releasing time to care. It involves a systematic and inclusive approach to improving the reliability, safety and efficiency of care delivery.[6] The programme is based on establishing good foundations which are (i) 'Knowing how we are doing' by developing ward-based measures to support informed decision making; (ii) having a well-organised ward and; (iii) knowing the patient status at a glance, which means having information to improve communication, patient experience and patient flow. Building on this foundation, a series of key ward processes can be examined – these include: meals, medicines, admission, planned discharge, shift handovers and patient hygiene. patient observation, nursing procedures and ward rounds.

I began by introducing governance and smart working processes, with the examples introduced highlighting that safe and effective care is closely bound up in efficient and effective ways of working. In some quarters patients have to fit into existing services, but current thinking is towards developing patient-centred service design. Smart processes need governing and a business plan is the vehicle to translate ideas into practice. In the coffee break you will have a chance to explore this further.

Yours truly,
Cartmel

Coffee break: governance, smart working processes and the business plan

Having considered the patient journey and the configuration of services around it, try following the method of lean thinking to identify where you think waste can be reduced.

1   Lean thinking

> • Map out the service user journey for your service.
>
> • Identify the participants, processes and resources associated with that journey.
>
> • Adopt a 'Lean Thinking' approach and identify examples of the types of waste in the journey.
>
> • Having identified some areas of waste think how they could be addressed and translated into action steps of change?

2   Business plans to translate ideas into practice

Having identified process development needs you need to think about how all the participants will 'buy into' the proposed change. One method is to specify the details of these changes in a business plan. The format for a business case is a variation on a theme and might have a particular house style but should include the following:

• An executive summary

This is a necessary synopsis of the key points of a business case on which the reader will make judgments about your business-based ideas from this section alone. You will want your reader to carefully consider rather than swiftly judge and discard your business plan – so making this informative, interesting and concise is paramount, being no more than two pages. It should include highlights from each section of the rest of the document – from the key features of the business opportunity through to the elements of the financial forecasts.

- A short description of the business opportunity
  Who you are, what you propose to offer, why and who will be benefited.
  Explain who is involved, perhaps with a paragraph on each individual including relevant experience and qualifications, together with their role in the organisation. You need to demonstrate that your management team has the right balance of skills, drive and experience to enable your plan to succeed.
- People involved
  Give details of your workforce in terms of total numbers and by department. Spell out what work you plan to do internally and if you plan to outsource any work. Other useful figures might be sales or profit per employee, average salaries, employee retention rates and productivity. Your plan should also outline any recruitment or training schemes, including timescales and costs.
    It is vital to be realistic about the commitment and motivation of your staff, and spell out any plans to improve or maintain staff morale.
- Your communication and implementation plan
  How you communicate or sell the proposal to staff and how you propose to implement the idea.
- Your management team and personnel
  Your credentials and the staff skill portfolio required to deliver the plan.
- Your operations
  Your premises, production facilities, management information systems and IT.
- Financial forecasts
  This section represents the plan in numbers.

Thus, a business plan might be a way of formalising planned change into an achievable and resourced trajectory. Finally, spend some time exploring clinical governance as a method of implementing systems management within a healthcare organisation.

3 Clinical governance
  Why clinical governance? Why do you think that we need clinical governance models and what pre-dated these in clinical services? Why did former health service arrangements need to change in the UK? An insight can be gained from the historical account included in Palmer's (2002) article.[1]
    A definition of clinical governance – Quality services arrayed around the patient journey require governing to ensure that harmony and synergies serve the chief purpose. Clinical governance is the system through which organisations 'are accountable for continuously improving the quality of

their services and safeguarding high standards of care, by creating an environment in which clinical excellence will flourish'.[2]

The Royal College of Nursing described it as 'the mechanism by which the public can be assured that NHS organisations have comprehensive and robust systems in place for continuously improving the quality of their services and safeguarding high standards of clinical care. It is the framework through which all the components of quality, including patient and public involvement, are brought together and placed high on the agenda of each organisation.'[3]

Representing clinical governance – One means of representing this is the seven pillars of clinical governance model developed by the NHS Clinical Governance Support team. In this model the apex of governance is partnership between the patient and the professional in decisions about treatment and care. The seven pillars are clinical effectiveness, clinical audit, risk management, patient experience, communication, resource management and learning. A different version of a governance model can be found in an Australian publication at www.safetyandquality.health.wa.gov.au.[4]

Having completed some exploration of governance, now turn your attention to workforce development and the people who make these processes work.

LETTER 3:   GOVERNANCE AND WORKFORCE DEVELOPMENT

Dear Marie,

If systems governance makes for a safe and effective care, it is the people who operate those systems that promote stable operation. However, in times of economic difficulty a response to making economic savings often involves workforce reduction. Whilst staff represents an easily identifiable major budgetary factor in terms of units of cost, is such a reduction a wise step? Granted, I have heard executives support their view that a health service is not an employment agency (in favour of reductions when necessary), but in another breath proudly assert that its greatest assets are people. Can both positions hold true? One day perhaps you too might face this decision-making dilemma, but it might not be so according to how you regard people. Indeed, valuing people is not always evident in the way in which they are seen to be treated in the workplace. So I propose to explore this with you, as it will certainly be a feature of your management work if not now, then certainly at some future point. What follows is an anecdote about workforce reduction based on an event that happened a few years ago.

A unit manager decided that it would make economic sense to remove sisters' posts and rely on senior staff nurses to oversee night duty teams. A year-long consultation ensued between staff, employers and the unions that culminated in the senior management's decision prevailing and subsequently over 3 years senior staff nurses oversaw the night shifts. It became evident, although anticipated long before, that the loss of experienced and mature staff on night duty would impact on care management and liaison with other professionals. This happened and ultimately led to appointment of night nurse practitioners – sisters under another name, and a useful device to save face for the manager who made the original decision.

What might this tell us? Employment has rules that govern terms and conditions; there is due process, representation, economic factors shaping decision making, short-termism in those decisions and human impact of decisions that are made. Overall, it also highlights continuing change surrounding service delivery. My question to you Marie is whether change has to be at the expense of people? The saying that 'a new broom sweeps clean' is common wisdom based on a synthesis of experience that a new manager often casts the existing staff as 'old guard' and makes claims that 'new blood' is needed to inject fresh vigour and ideas into the service. Circumstances can be utilised or even 'created' to make an underpinning business case as to the need to reduce staff. The merits of doing this can be debated and perhaps sometimes some organisations need to renew their 'mindset', and this is the only shortcut to achieving that. Even government tries a parallel approach when casting competing parties' policies in a particularly jaded light to construct a case for necessary change. Likewise, failing schools can have a management team imported to set them back on a path of measurable achievement.

Workforce planning is about getting the right people with the right skills in the right place at the right time to deliver the planned service without compromising quality. In some ways this might appear as a mechanical approach in which required roles are identified, and the round peg is acquired to fit the round hole. This sounds fine in theory but needs to be tempered with a broader view that includes existing staff whom you might 'inherit' on assuming management responsibility for a service. Indeed, your most likely scenario will include developing the shape of an existing service rather than commissioning something entirely new.

Your thinking around workforce planning can be developed by asking a series of questions in relation to the model given. What is the demand for healthcare services in the host community? This will drive considerations of service design and allow analysis of the demand for such services. Next, what resources are available to provide a service to meet this demand? What type of workforce is needed? The ideal can be mapped against the existing staff resources to decide what additions and changes might be needed. A plan can be devised to provide the workforce for the new service that combines new staff appointments and existing staff development.

A six step methodology similar to this description has been published in the NHS Healthcare Workforce Portal.[1] These six steps are to define the plan, including a description of what is required; identify forces for change – any workforce development involves change and so for it to succeed it's necessary to work out what is likely to support or resist this. A force field analysis is useful to identify which ones can be controlled and which cannot. The term 'lever' is given to forces that exert change and some will be amenable to control such as training, pay, skill mix, service delivery, and investment in new processes and technologies. Other external factors are beyond direct control. One way of identifying these forces is by using a fishbone diagram (this is referred to as a causal analysis). A PEST analysis (political, social, economic and technological) is also useful for examining the context of these levers. Identify the demand for staff to provide the service. Next, the demand in terms of numbers and skills of staff needed to provide a service has to be determined. Once completed, the supply has to be identified, which involves assessing the numbers of people with the required skills. If this supply is insufficient, other options such as skill mix need to be considered. The supply and demand relationship shapes decision making – if the supply of the staff cannot be achieved then in theory the demand will have to be reduced – but in practice this is not always in equilibrium and undersupply is made up from a reserve army of agency or bank staff. The risk to safe and effective service delivery increases as the supply decreases. It is at this stage that throughput of staff must be examined to reduce attrition and attract new applicants.

One way of evaluating service risk is to identify supply gaps and determine the level of threat to service delivery. A case in point might be a shortage of clinical experts. A role mapping exercise can also be undertaken to map the required skill requirement against the existing workforce to determine who could be offered development to meet emerging requirements.

Finally, there is implementation of a plan within an agreed budget along with periodic progress reviews. The success and sustainability of the plan will partially depend on steps taken to promote retention, perhaps with training and development, and offering opportunities to develop new skills and roles.

If workforce development is about making the best use of available resources and procuring what is required, then it becomes apparent that investment is also needed to ensure competent management performance. We can mechanically assess and plan, but some of these problems associated with threats to service continuity would be alleviated if the value of the resources was truly appreciated. I refer to this as intellectual capital – the combined value of knowledge and experience in the local setting. Losing staff is more than names on the payroll and in your coffee break take time to consider workforce development in your own setting and the consequences of the loss of intellectual capital.

Yours truly,
Cartmel

Coffee break: intellectual and social capital

1   Recognising change

When you manage staff effectively their experience of work can be fulfilling and productive, which in turn contributes to workforce stability. This has an impact on service quality. This investment is not to be underestimated, but change can threaten this stability. Indeed, it can be a catalyst that prompts staff to leave employment, which is sometimes euphemistically called 'career development.' Just as the patient has a journey, so do staff. In this coffee break consider the challenges to workforce stability in your workplace.

- Revisit the staff journey from initial interest in a post through to their leaving employment.

- What is the rate of staff turnover in your unit over the past year?

- How does this compare to the whole organisation over the same period?

- What changes are impacting on your workplace?

- How is this impacting on the local workforce?

- Draw a force field diagram to analyse factors supporting and resisting change in your workplace. Which factors could be controlled to promote staff retention (workforce stability)? Which factors cannot be controlled and what are the implications of these for you as a manager?

- How does knowing about controllable and uncontrollable factors inform your approach to managing staff and promoting team stability?

2 The impact of staff turnover
   When a staff member leaves their post, the unit loses more than just a person who undertook so many hours of work per week. It loses local knowledge, experience and expertise. I call this intellectual capital. Additionally, it loses a part of a social network, a character with an interpersonal skill set, a colleague, even a friend of the staff team – this I call social capital. Whilst no one is indispensable, a team can encounter a sense of loss, and tangibly so when a staff member retires or even dies in post.

- In terms of professional decision making how would you describe the value of the intellectual capital in your unit?

- What effect might the loss of intellectual capital have on professional decision making and patient safety?

- How does loss of social capital weaken the stability of the workforce?

- How do your reflections on intellectual and social capital inform your approach to managing staff?

Decision making and resource management

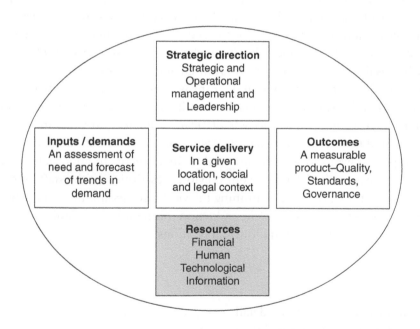

LETTER 1: GOVERNANCE AND THE STAFF JOURNEY: RECOGNISING THE INVESTMENT

Dear Marie,

You wrote recently asking whether or not staff should be described as a resource. The answer depends on your standpoint. If you take a 'business' approach that the workforce is engaged in production, which in our case is service provision, then the means of production is a social organisation that draws on a range of technologies to achieve its goals. In times of surplus, when supply outstrips service demand, staff are made redundant. When demand outstrips supply a reserve army of temporary labour (such as agency staff) can be hired. I'm not convinced that labelling people as a resource is helpful as it has connotations of people as a commodity. However, when a resource is valued beyond its function (employment to fulfil a given role) it can have positive connotations. This type of valuing recognises investment in the social and intellectual capital of the workforce – and we are wise when we do not neglect this. There is no guarantee that treating people fairly but firmly will ensure workforce stability, but it does establish and endorse ground rules that operate within the workplace to benefit all staff. These are based on employment law, operational policies and protocols, and are enacted through the behaviour of managers. There is a parable about a good shepherd who cares for his sheep and keeps them safe, whereas the hireling cares only for himself and as a consequence the sheep are prey to outside dangers. You will find a canvas depicting this by William Holman Hunt (1851) in the Manchester Art Gallery entitled The Hireling Shepherd – look it up on the internet and you will see what I mean.[1] Therefore, the relevance of this to managing staff is to recognise and protect workforce investment. After all, any good business person wants to see a return on their investment. To appreciate the scope of this investment let's pick up on your previous description of the staff journey.

I will start at the point of determining the workforce requirement, moving onto recruitment, selection, appointment, induction, probation, appraisal and development, leaving employment and industrial relations.

Workforce requirement

Once this has been agreed, the detail of a given post can be clarified. Whether it's an existing post or not, a role description will need to be written or revised. This describes what the person will actually do. The role specification identifies the knowledge, skills and education required to be able to do the job. It includes essential and desirable criteria. It might also be mapped against a knowledge and skills framework to support the rationale for aligning the post to a specific pay band. To expand your learning, about writing role descriptions consider what you would expect to see in a role description. How much supporting information should be provided about the organisation, and what is an applicant likely to ask about the role and employer?

Job advertisement, where to publicise, web

Previously I have touched on workforce planning involving deciding whether the pool of labour exists either from internal development opportunities or from outside of the organisation. These factors will inform decisions about the cost and place of advertising, such as on a website, in a local newspaper or in a professional journal to access the intended audience. A specialist practitioner might be attracted from further afield, whereas a part-time domestic worker would typically be someone local. The advertisement also has to comply with legal obligations, including equal opportunities legislation. You need to be aware of what can and cannot be stated in an advertisement, and you would not be able to discriminate on grounds of gender or religion unless special circumstances are permitted. For more details check out the Equality and Human Rights Commission web pages.[2]

The advertisement will also answer job seekers' questions. These include: job title, location, salary, employer, work environment and salary, and a contact number, email or web address (URL) for enquiries. By adding a note about key requirements, job seekers can determine whether or not they qualify for the post and so only those who fit the essential criteria should ultimately apply. This could save on filtering out ineligible applications later on.

Application packs

Assuming the job seeker requires more information, the application pack can be provided as a web download. Alternatively, this might be managed by postal application from a human resources officer within the organisation. Details also need to be provided about the application process, closure date and how unsuccessful applicants will know if they are successful or not – typically a statement is made that if applicants have not had a response after a specified number of weeks they can assume that they have not been selected for interview.

Applications will be reviewed according to explicit criteria, normally the essential criteria on the role specification. The selection of candidates needs to be made on the basis of having met the essential criteria. There could be several reasons why you do not get any applications – the terms and conditions offered might not be competitive, the market could have a glut of jobs, the staff pool might be small, the service might have a poor reputation or the advertisement could have been published in the wrong 'market place' or at the wrong time.

Interview

Assuming that there are sufficient applicants, and it is a judgement call about how many are enough, you will invite candidates to interview. The letter will include details of venue, date and time together with evidence that must be brought to the interview such as professional certificates. At this stage you need to be clear about the way in which the interview will generate answers to your questions to inform your appointment decision. If the post requires competency in a particular skill you might include that as part of the interview process (e.g. a typing exercise or problem-solving scenario). Once you are clear about this you can invite candidates for interview and instruct them to prepare for specific tests or presentations. Some interviews last 2 or 3 days and involve a series of psychometric tests, exercises, written assessments and interviews. It all depends on whom you want to employ and what purpose the interview will serve in making the right decision. The application form should tell you the applicant's curriculum vitae – their professional knowledge, skills and experience, along with a personal statement about why they are interested in the post.

A date is set for the interviews – some application processes allow the candidate to book the most convenient interview slot online and confirm their attendance. If the candidate is travelling some distance you might offer terms for reimbursement of travel and accommodation. It is helpful to accommodate the travelling arrangements of candidates who have to travel some distance to attend by giving them a later interview slot. An interview panel is also arranged, typically comprising a service manager, team member and human resources representative. In the meantime, close to the event the interview panel will have a copy of the application forms and agreement will be reached on the questions that will be asked, by whom and in which order.

On the day of the interview ensure that the candidates have a clear place to report to and somewhere to wait, along with provision of nearby facilities (refreshments and toilets). An administrator might make a copy of the original qualification certificates and evidence of residency, work permit and birth certificate.

The actual interview needs to be conducted in a way that puts the candidate at ease, and a simple way to achieve this is to open the interview by explaining the process and then letting the candidate explain a little about themselves. Following this, each of the interview panel team will ask questions about their agreed focus. Finally, the candidate should be given the opportunity to ask any questions of the panel.

The offer and appointment

After the interview the panel will adjourn to make its decision based on discussion and a transparent scoring system for each candidate's performance. This decision will be communicated to the successful candidate, usually by telephone. If the candidate's acceptance of a job cannot be confirmed immediately (perhaps time is needed to negotiate terms and conditions) a point of closure will be agreed. Assuming agreement, a formal job offer letter is sent from the human resources department. At this stage references, if not already taken up, are obtained as well as a criminal records bureau check and a pre-employment medical examination arranged through an occupational health department. The offer letter will state that employment is subject to satisfactory completion of these requirements. Following this, a date to commence employment will be issued along with instructions about the local arrangements for the first day.

Induction

I can recall different induction experiences that demonstrated a real lack of forethought on how a new staff member would integrate into the team. Some amounted to a tour of the ward and sight of a file of policies before launching into shift work. An induction should include local service orientation, mandatory health and safety training, allocation of a mentor from the local team and an induction plan. Some organisations have an induction pack that the new staff member can work through, including reading relevant documents and meeting staff relevant to their work. Large organisations have corporate induction events led by senior staff at set times during the year and require new starters to attend these as they arise.

Probation

Following commencement of employment a new staff member has to satisfactorily complete a probation period. The criteria will be set to facilitate goal achievement and subsequent sign off at the period's end. It's common practice to allow 3 months or longer depending on the training and skill sets required to undertake the role. Throughout this time the employee will be made aware of the performance and behavioural standards expected. Required training should be provided and supervision meetings must be planned to monitor progress. This probation period can be extended if the employer has concerns about the employee's performance and will be regularly reviewed. A meeting should take place prior to the end of the probation period to review whether the necessary standards have been achieved and to proceed to a formal 'sign off' indicating successful completion of probation. This is also communicated to the human resources department as it has contractual implications and a letter is normally sent to the employee to notify them of successful completion of their probation. If, however, the employer believes the employee is unlikely to attain the necessary standards, even though they have been provided with all the necessary support and training, a decision can be made to terminate the contract. Naturally, you would liaise with your human resources staff to verify the exact details of this process.

Preceptorship

Preceptorship is provided to help newly registered individuals make the transition from being a student to an accountable practitioner. Its aim is to facilitate practise in accordance with their professional code and to develop confidence in their competence as a registered professional.

To facilitate this, a new registrant should have protected learning time and access to a preceptor. They will hold regular meetings with the staff member, take steps to facilitate their knowledge and skill acquisition, and give positive feedback on aspects of good performance. They will also make the staff member aware of the standards, competencies, or objectives that have been set so that they are clear about what is required to be achieved. A preceptor should also provide objective feedback on aspects of performance that are a cause for concern and assist the staff member to develop a plan of action to remedy these.

Appraisal

Management supervision is about working with the employee to ensure that they have what is necessary to do their job. It also ensures a feedback loop where the line manager has information about the job in order to be able to support the employee. In this way, the line manager has an opportunity to address any problems that may arise. The management supervision process involves an appraisal (or performance review) during which goals are set for the year. This is followed by a sequence of planned meetings to evaluate progress. This culminates in an end of year review. Some roles have performance management targets linked to rewards. In summary, it has the following features:

1   It is a formal hierarchical yet enabling and supportive process rather than a directive process. It gives the supervisee the opportunity to attain realistic agreed goals. It therefore has clear definition for both participants.
2   It aims to improve the working performance of the supervisee. There will be a supervision contract detailing the purpose, preparation and expectations of both participants.
3   The supervisee will have time to review concerns as well as to evaluate and assess achievement in the context of a private and confidential discussion. Management supervision is normally recorded and kept on the supervisee's personal file. It is confidential to the two parties involved but may be accessed as part of a disciplinary investigation. The agenda can be set in advance or negotiated at the start of the session.
4   The supervisor will be informed of the supervisee's needs to facilitate professional and personal development. It therefore involves developing a working relationship, and this implies the use of skills including coaching, challenging and negotiating as required.

Development

Development is linked to individual appraisal goals. The workforce is diverse and individuals will be at different stages of their working life, with different skills, experiences, maturity and interests. It is the remit of the manager to harness this diversity and to work with it so as to enhance the resource in order to benefit the purposes of the service and the participants themselves. This sounds fine in theory but is more complicated in practice. Limited resources shape staff development through negotiation on funding and time investment necessary to achieve goals. This might not match staff expectations and is exacerbated if there is a perception or evidence of favouritism. It is best to have an explicit agreement about how development will be supported. Some workplaces have a pecking order – this year it is agreed that some staff members can share the development resource between them, next year a different set of staff. That can work if the team is stable and in post for several years, and all agree to the ground rules. Some workplaces have a per capita allowance for development that colleagues can opt to donate to others to use so that a greater resource is available to attend conferences or courses. Another way to support staff development includes drawing resources into the unit through successful applications to funding bodies for set projects. Apart from funding, other means of staff development include making links to local networks, symposia and colloquiums. Additionally, development should also encompass social events, which can be organisationally led, such as staff development weeks, staff fairs, learning and teaching weeks, and national day events as well as local initiatives such as sharing a buffet lunch after a working meeting, having a team social at on-site cafes or dress down Fridays. In summary, the employee should be offered a broad employment package that supports personal, social and professional development, and each organisation will have its own way of addressing this.

Leaving

Workforce stability is to be desired but external factors and internal dynamics can and do threaten this, leading predictably to staff turnover. People leave their employment for a variety of reasons, be it planned (e.g. retirement, voluntary severance, ill health, career change) or otherwise. Whatever the reason is, there are at least two actions that should be taken. First is to be generous and show a token of appreciation for the contribution that the person made whilst employed. People who leave feeling aggrieved or unappreciated will give a particular account of their workplace experience and this can be counterproductive. I have known staff with over a decade's service leave their post and the employer not provide a formal event to mark the event or express their thanks to the staff member. That situation is lamentable and reveals the indifference of local managers and their seniors. With social networking on the rise, it could threaten the image of and the trust placed in the service.

Next you should seek to understand why people leave. A formal step is to hold an exit interview, but this is not guaranteed to elicit the real reasons why someone has chosen to leave. Far better though, to be an involved manager who knows their staff. To use the analogy of a farmer, there is a proverb about dealing with the welfare of people that states, 'Be sure you know the condition of your flocks, give careful attention to your herds'.[3]

Next you should consider the effect on the team of someone leaving – sometimes staff mourns the loss of a respected colleague. Old alliances and relationships have to readjust, and personal investment is needed to help staff work through a period of change and to focus in an engaged way on the organisation's goals. This is particularly the case where staff has been invited to take early retirement or voluntary severance. Once staff have had their motivation dented as a result of the way in which they perceived the organisation is treating them and an element of cynicism has crept in, it takes real labour to lead them back to a position of trust. Some never do, and develop survival and coping strategies that mediate the direct effect of the organisation on their daily activities. Part of that skill set is to outwit their manager as if they were playing a chess game whilst remaining just within the letter of employment 'rules'. In this way they regain some control over their working life as a means of regulating the impact of change.

Industrial relations

When working relationships break down we find ourselves in a territory that siphons resources away from investment in the service. Trades unions exist to uphold the rights of the employee and work to support them whenever these are threatened. As a manager you would want to be fair and act within the law. You would not bully or harass staff, nor discriminate on grounds of colour, ethnicity, gender, age, religion or disability. You yourself would not, but others sometimes do, and so it is necessary for recognised procedures to be used. Staff can raise matters informally on a one-to-one basis, perhaps in management supervisions or call special meetings. Sometimes the other party will not be aware that their behaviour or actions are causing a problem, and issues can be resolved at this point through discussion and clarification.

Another informal mechanism is mediation that is undertaken without any admission of wrong doing by any party, and without preventing any opportunity to pursue formal action. This is a voluntary process in which a third-party helps others to resolve their difficulties. It can be used to resolve conflict, treat people fairly, create realistic workable agreements, and work to change behaviour that is creating difficulty for an employee. The process of mediation facilitates opportunities to speak and listen, exchange feelings and ideas, and negotiate solutions.

An employee can submit a grievance in writing to their line manager unless it involves them, in which case it is submitted to the line manager's manager. They will invite the employee to a meeting as soon as possible, normally within 2 weeks of receipt of the written grievance (although this timescale can be varied by mutual agreement) to examine the issues raised.

The employee may be accompanied by a trade union representative or fellow employee at all stages of this formal process. The grievance is heard by a manager who is at least at the level of the manager causing the grievance. The process involves meeting the person presenting the grievance and seeking a view on how they think it could be settled. The attendees at a grievance meeting would be the chair, the employee who raised the grievance and, if chosen, a trade union representative or nominated friend. A member of the human resources team will provide advice and guidance to the chair, and will keep a record of the meeting.

The chair will look at the matters that have given rise to the hearing, including the reasonableness of the behaviour and decision making of all parties, including any previous informal processes, and will consider all the information that has been presented. They might ask questions during any grievance meeting and can adjourn to allow further investigations to take place if there is good reason to do so. The reasons for any adjournment have to be given to all parties to the grievance verbally on the day of the adjournment and confirmed in writing within a specified period. The employee will normally be notified of the outcome of the meeting in writing by human resources within 1 week of the hearing. That letter will also include notification of the right to appeal against the decision.

In all cases, the employee should seek advice from an appropriate source such as an human resources officer or a trade union representative.

What can we learn from this? Knowing and working within employment law and organisational policy is a safeguard against inadvertently disadvantaging a staff member. Knowing how to manage people effectively will alert you to emerging issues long before they erupt into tension within the manager–employee relationship.

Well Marie, the staff journey is rich and varied, and the above has highlighted the importance of management skills at different stages of the staff journey. These can be categorised into two domains – one about knowing processes, procedures, legal and policy frameworks. The other is about knowing people, the diversity of your workforce and how they act and react to events. To provide good services we need to not only manage robust systems but also effectively manage people. Competent governance of the staff journey is essential to maximise the available expenditure on workforce planning and development. The process is enacted by competent people who can bring positive management skills to the workplace. In your coffee break take time to explore and reflect on your own management style.

Yours truly,
Cartmel

Coffee break: governance and management style

1 Managing staff – being an encourager
You might have heard the light-hearted saying that 'the beatings will continue until morale improves.' Whilst humorous, it is like the story of a donkey pulling

a cart – the driver beats the donkey if it does not move whilst dangling a carrot in front of the donkey to entice it forward. This carrot and stick approach might describe an organisational approach to workforce management – stick by threatened sanctions and carrots through staff development opportunities.

- To what extent can you detect this in your own organisation?
- If this is the case, how could it be altered?
- Do staff need to have boundaries that when crossed trigger sanctions?
- Is it possible to attain a state within a team where the boundary of sanctions is not needed?
- Where do disciplinary rules fit into a carrot and stick analogy?

2   Managing staff – disciplinary action
Managers have to deal with disciplinary matters, and disciplinary procedure is designed to deal with situations where behaviour falls below an acceptable standard. Look up your organisation's disciplinary policy and procedure. Particularly note the different types of disciplinary offence and the levels of response as well as the sanction that is applied.

Compare your local organisation's disciplinary procedure with advice provided on the Chartered Institute of Personnel and Development (CIPD) website 'The HR and development website'.[1] Next, compare your local organisation's guidance with that provided by the advisory, conciliation and arbitration service (ACAS). ACAS provides information on grievance procedures and the disciplinary process. ACAS's purpose is stated as: 'We aim to improve organisations and working life through better employment relations. We help with employment relations by supplying up-to-date information, independent advice and high quality training, and working with employers and employees to solve problems and improve performance'.[2]

Look at the following examples of disciplinary action, and having studied them how do these inform your vigilance as a manager to recognise breaches of discipline? What can you do to develop your vigilance to protect the integrity of the service?

Hospital sacks senior manager over stolen laptop

- Health chiefs in Colchester fired a senior manager who lost confidential records on thousands of patients after his hospital laptop was stolen[3,4]

Press release: Police in hospital deaths inquiry[5]

- Nurse dismissed after four patients die in intensive care unit

Case studies of recent NHS fraud cases[6]

- Timesheet fraud, stealing drugs, forgery, failing to carry out safety checks

3 Managing staff – which style?

If effective management of the organisation's most valuable asset is essential, what approach will you take? In many management texts you will read about democratic, autocratic, consultative and laissez-faire management styles. Your management style may lead to greater motivation and productivity from your staff. However, it is not as simple as just 'picking' a style as individual personalities and characteristics influence this. Read the following summaries and consider the extent to which any of these describe your style. Can your management style alter according to the situation? If so, what factors shape your choice of a different style? Do staff prefer a particular management style – or is it impossible to generalise?

Democratic management style

A democratic manager delegates authority to their staff so that they take the responsibility to complete the task given to them. Staff will complete their tasks using their own work methods. Through including staff in decision making it engenders ownership and enhances motivation, which has an impact on the quality of decision making and work outcomes. On the other hand a democratic management style can actually slow decision making due to the need for consultation.

Autocratic management style

An autocratic manager dictates orders to their staff and makes decisions without any consultation. They prefer control and quick decisions so that work is usually completed on time. However, because of this approach staff motivation can decrease and staff turnover increases.

Consultative management style

A consultative style is a combination of the above two. The manager will ask for views and opinions from their staff, allowing them to feel involved, but will ultimately make the final decision.

Laissez-faire management style

A laissez-faire manager sets the tasks and gives staff complete freedom to complete the task as they see fit with minimal involvement. The manager acts as a coach and provides information if required. It has the benefit of staff ownership and development, and may lead to improved motivation. Its drawback can be that with little direction staff may feel lost and not reach their goals.

LETTER 2: MANAGING INFORMATION AND COMMUNICATION

Dear Marie,

Have you thought how your management style is related to the way in which you handle and share information? Management decision making relies on information and a structure through which it can be accessed and shared. Having formal and informal aspects, this system must be effective for an organisation to function effectively. However, information is not value free, and as previously mentioned, some managers regulate information disclosure – deciding what and whom to share it with, thus creating divisions within teams amongst those who are informed and those who are excluded. You can address this by identifying formal and informal channels, the value of information as a resource and identify skills needed as an information worker.

So what are the formal information channels? You can work out the answer to this by referring to the organisational model. Each element needs interconnecting links that can be equated to channels in the formal information organisation. Each link between elements represents an agreed way of sharing information. It follows that there will be information about delivery (the central element), the strategic (corporate) function, resource management, monitoring demand and output measures. This occurs in a particular setting and there will be a link between the executive (or agreed representative), external stakeholders and the public.

Informal communication flows between networks. This is via alliances and relationships that transcend formal structures and operate outside them. The grapevine or rumour mill is often grounded in uninformed analysis rather than evidence, but none the less is potent. Whether these networks are regarded as a threat or merely a feature of social interactions, they are the 'soft' side of 'hard' systems within an organisation.

Usually organisations will have a corporate information area (whether on an intranet site or paper publications). It will typically explain the organisational structure and the links between each of its sections, the relationships between different sections and the executive management team. Allied to this will often be a communications strategy that articulates the agreed methods, frequency and domains of external and internal communication. This typically includes details about systems, responsiveness and publicity.

Systems details include internal and external structures, procedures and practices to enable a two-way flow of information. Responsive communication utilises procedures, policies and practices that is open, transparent and accountable. Publicity details are about promoting the organisation's achievements (whether in reports, league tables or star ratings) in a way that promotes public confidence and engagement. In this way the communications strategy projects an image to the public that faithfully represents its aims, objectives and values. Examples of corporate communication are found in annual reports, press releases and newsletters.

Robust communication is vital and is a recurring weakness in many organisations. It needs to be reciprocal from the top downwards and bottom upwards.

Top-down communication includes circulating meeting minutes, road shows, intranet publications, emails, webcasts, bulletins and letters included with wage statements. Bottom-up communication occurs through local meetings feeding upwards to departmental managers and executive levels. Anonymous feedback can also be captured through staff suggestion boxes and surveys.

A communications policy also reveals power and positional authority within an organisation. In contrast to informal networks (the grapevine) that circumvent formal information channels. In political circles information is deliberately leaked (e.g. to newspaper reporters) for various reasons, including malicious, subversive and maverick behaviour and also public interest. This boosts newspaper sales but can be illegal and break professional codes associated with confidentiality and protection of personal information, damaging the organisation's reputation and public trust in it. Guidance is published to advise staff of the boundaries and consequences of unauthorised information disclosure. The following example highlights the gravity of the consequences:

Disclosure of confidential information[1]

Employees must not during the course of their employment or after its termination, use or disclose to any other person or institution information made available to them during their employment with the trust, except in pursuance of the authorised business of the trust. Such information includes details relating to identifiable patients, members of staff or the business/commercial interests of the trust. Business/commercial interests normally involve information, which if disclosed to a competitor would be liable to cause significant or real harm to the trust. A breach of such confidentiality will result in serious disciplinary action including dismissal, being taken. This duty of confidentiality applies to staff representatives of trade unions or staff associations.

Well Marie, information is vital but has to be governed. Your decision making will require an awareness of the Freedom of Information Act, and in connection with disclosure it is worth checking how public interest is interpreted.

Yours,
Cartmel

Coffee break: freedom of information and communications strategy

In this coffee break begin by looking through the Freedom of Information Act (FOIA): that is accessible via The Information Commissioner's Office (ICO)[1] and consider the following:

- When is information 'caught' by the FOIA?

- What is the duty to confirm or deny the existence of information?

- What is exempted from the FOI?

- What is the Public Interest test? Refer to the Freedom of Information Act Awareness Guidance No 3 The Public Interest Test 1. March 2007 ICO.

- Look through the list of absolute and qualified exemptions in the act.

Whilst the FOIA deals with specifics regarding decisions about disclosure, a broader debate surrounds the place of the dividing line between disclosure and non disclosure of information.

- In terms of external communications what should the public know and not know about a service and its performance?

- How would a senior manager decide what the public should be told?

- What process does your local organisation stipulate that should be followed when making a disclosure?

- Are there advantages to keeping information from the public?

- Why could it be beneficial?

- What problems are caused by withholding information from the public?

- What criteria should be used to make decisions about disclosure?

Now turn your study to familiarising yourself with examples of communication strategies. Undertake a simple web search (try typing: 'NHS Trust Communication strategy' into a search engine) and examine the aims and objectives of the strategies to note the commonality amongst them.

Here is an example of the way in which the aims of a communications strategy are presented:

Aims of the communications strategy[2]

1. To ensure internal and external audiences are well informed about what is happening within the Trust and its future developments;

2. To ensure key corporate messages are disseminated and understood;

3. To ensure staff and stakeholders are listened to, given the opportunity to voice opinions, and receive feedback on their views;

4. To provide clarity on who is responsible for ensuring communications are effective and coordinated;

5. To improve staff morale by listening and communicating more effectively;

6. To enhance the Trust's reputation.

LETTER 3: HEALTH INFORMATICS

Dear Marie,

So you have recently come across a real breach of confidentiality that has resulted in a disciplinary action. Well, that is interesting and serves to emphasise the importance of information governance. It conveniently directs our attention towards information management.

Health informatics is the current label for this field of work. Its origins are in the introduction of computers into healthcare from the 1960s in general practice, hospital laboratories, radiotherapy planning, in patient monitoring and hospital activity analysis. This emerging field that was initially called medical computing later became termed medical informatics as more general data recording and analysis was included. The term health informatics emerged as this activity extended in scope beyond hospitals. It is now a feature of modern healthcare with its nascent 'professionals' – information workers (or informaticians) having defined skill sets such as those in the NHS key skills framework (NHS KSF) according to their level of engagement with data.[1]

It has been defined as: 'The knowledge, skills and tools which enable information to be collected, managed, used and shared to support delivery of healthcare and to promote health'[2] and current practise is grounded in a cluster of legislation including: The Computer Misuse Act 1990; Data protection Act 1998; European Directive on Data Protection 1995 (directive 95/46/EC); Access to Health Records Act 1990; Freedom of Information Act 2000.

There is a difference between data and information. Data is the raw material that is processed to become information. Information allows descriptions of the 'what' (e.g. what the trend is) whilst knowledge is the understanding of how to use information (e.g. the trend is upwards) and an interpretation of its meaning. However, an information system is only as good as its data quality, which must be accurate, contemporaneous, and free from duplication and ambiguity so as to be fit for the purpose.

Informatics is also altering how service users approach healthcare decision making, so that the locus of decision control will be negotiated between professionals and themselves on a case-by-case basis. Public access to healthcare information also means that they will acquire information from a range of sources of differing quality, but not necessarily hold the same understanding about a given topic as a professional. This insight, however, will influence what service users seek from a consultation. Likewise, health professionals need to develop technology user skills so as to be able to access and critique a range of electronically hosted information.

Another impact on service user care is the introduction of an e-record to support direct patient care and enhance decision making via an effective means of multi-disciplinary communication. Furthermore, the e-record supports clinical audit, research, resource allocation, performance monitoring and service planning.

Information usage signifies change as new applications come 'online', such as electronic choose and book services, electronic prescription services, health records transfer between GPs, e-scheduling (e.g. in operating departments) and enhanced patient administration services. Whilst these offer practical support in service delivery, other developments can bring resources to local settings through virtual healthcare. This allows collaboration and information sharing about service users. Telecare allows remote physical monitoring of a person and mobile (mHealth) uses mobile devices to collect service user health data, perform real-time monitoring and even direct provision of care (via mobile telemedicine). Professional development can be enhanced by e-learning, which distributes education at a time, place and pace of the learner's choosing.

Well Marie, the information revolution is bringing rapid change to the workplace, and a skill set is needed to govern and use information. In your coffee break, take time to review local procedures surrounding information governance that are generic across all information workers. Then progress to consider the effectiveness of e-communication compared to other forms of communication. Perhaps you might find a paperless office a burden or a blessing.

Yours truly,
Cartmel

Coffee break: local procedures and information management

Take time to examine local information management procedures specifically focusing on the following:

- Data Protection Act
- Data security
- Passwords and patient identifiable data

Contemporary communication: what do you think?

I was at an exhibition recently at the War Museum North about 'Animals at war.' Prominent in one of the display cases was a stuffed pigeon and photographic illustrations of how these had message canisters attached to them. Aeroplane crews would release them during operations over enemy territory so that secure messages could be sent back to base. That was quite an ingenious yet simple formal communication system that proved to be functional. Other communication channels have included lamps (to send line of sight messages as a series of Morse code dots and dashes), radio, telephone and publications. Contemporary developments have included podcasts, blogs, wikis and networking sites (face book). The point is that there are different ways of formally communicating information either visually, verbally or in objects such as written text (by formal I mean in a planned and approved way). Access to such communication will include granting permission to receive the information and possessing the necessary skills and use of equipment – even using a telephone is a skill to be learnt, just as was caring for a carrier pigeon.

- What is your definition of effective communication?
- What is your definition of efficient communication?
- What steps can be taken to support effective electronic communication within your workplace?
- What are the enablers and barriers to supporting effective electronic communication in the workplace?
- How might you minimise these barriers?
- How will a paperless office enhance or impede your work?

Decision making and the service user journey

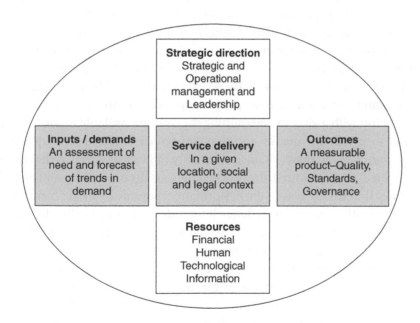

LETTER 1: THE SERVICE USER JOURNEY – HEALTH NEEDS ASSESSMENT

Dear Marie,

You comment that technology can deflect from maintaining a focus on service user care is pertinent. In order to help to maintain priorities we need to return to the service model that has the central feature of a service user journey as a trajectory ranging across it. This commences with need and demand arising from within the host community, proceeding through to access and use of service provision, and eventually leading to the point of exiting the service.

To understand service demand we need to have data about the health needs in the host community, trends in changing patterns of need and the way in which your particular service is situated to address some of these. Health needs assessment is a systematic method for reviewing the health issues facing a population, leading to agreeing priorities and allocating resources to improve health and reduce inequalities.

The relationship between the public and services can be understood as a purchaser-provider relationship; although a designated commissioning body might purchase care services on behalf of the host community. However, this is not always the case, and individuals can purchase their own healthcare services, such as surgical treatment or home care nursing either by paying for it themselves or through an insurance scheme.

Commissioning services requires an assessment of the host population's health needs, and will include community-based views about health needs and their priorities in contrast to professionals' perspectives. The commissioner will appraise the information with a view to determining the options available to meet identified needs, and to specify the quality and levels of service required. Providers have to tender for contracts and these will include quality indicators as well as the cost in the package offered. Once procured, the provider delivers the care service and establishes the measures that will be part of the performance monitoring in the contract.

You will recall from an earlier letter how a definition of health directly influences how health needs are identified. Assessment of demand might be thought of as an alternative to health need, but these are not the same. Whilst there are people needing particular short-term interventions and others requiring long-term care, underlying patterns of health status in the host community could be hidden by focusing purely on demand. Furthermore, perpetuating historical patterns of service provision can obscure the need to reconfigure services to address community health needs. Specialist healthcare services, whilst admirable, may reflect the interests of a clinical team and their success in drawing resources, but not be warranted by local healthcare need. However, there will always be an element of this – a provider will have local clusters of expertise and possibly research activity of national or international repute. This does make for leading edge service development. Service development decision making has therefore to accommodate its strengths and consider how to work with internal diversity, growing some aspects, reducing others and generating new services. In short, there will be factors that preserve the historical shape of service provision and sometimes there will only be incremental changes within block contracts rather than radical alterations.

So how are health needs actually assessed? You could work this out by asking questions about the profile of the population, what they consider their health needs to be, what are the impacts of these health needs on that population and which need is to be prioritised for action along with what actions are required. There are different variants of approaches to health needs assessment – The National Institute for Health and Clinical Excellence NICE, for example, provides a five-step process.[1]

Step 1 is about getting started and ranges questions about what population, who needs to be involved, what resources are required and what the risks are? Step 2 considers how to identify health priorities, including population profiling, gathering data, perceptions of needs, identifying and assessing health conditions and determinant factors. Step 3 is about assessing health priorities for action and requires choosing health conditions and determinant factors with the most significant size and severity impact. Effective and acceptable interventions and actions are determined, leading to step 4, which is planning for change. This includes stating the aims of intervention and action planning. As with a business plan that I mentioned in a previous letter, action plans need to be checked for progress via monitoring and evaluation. The final step, 5, is 'moving on and review.' Following the cycle of assessment, plan intervention and evaluation, learning needs to take place to decide what the impact was and to consider how this informs future decisions.

Whilst benefits of this process include community engagement and partnership working, challenges exist around power and politics amongst stakeholders, on agreement about what health needs are and how to measure these with problems of gaining access to the host population to gather data in the first place. Health needs assessment is not a neutral subject to which you apply a mechanical assessment tool. The key decisions lie with those who determine the meaning of health and so devise corresponding health measurements, because in the final analysis these shape how the health of the population is understood and so informs the nature of services required. Given the strength of some stakeholders, there may be a reduced community representation about their own health needs and so they themselves may have little meaningful impact on action plans about service provision. So how would you go about undertaking a health needs assessment?

Yours,
Cartmel

Coffee break: health needs assessment

This coffee break can be spent reviewing the guidance provided to undertake a health needs assessment and then seeing the detail of real examples. You might need a refill by the time you get to the end of this!

- The process of health needs assessment

> The process of health needs assessment is provided in more detail in this NICE publication: Summary: Health needs assessment at a glance.[1]
>
> Read the guide and then inspect a real example of a health needs assessment. There are many that can be easily accessed on the internet – one specific example is Swansea's Health, Social Care and Well-Being (HSCWB) Needs assessment (2007).[2]
>
> Note particularly the health map and determinants of health and well-being (page 5). How do these determinants compare with those used in your locality?
>
> Social capital is mentioned in the above report – (page 31). What similarities can you see between this and the social and intellectual capital within the staff group in your service? How does defining social and intellectual capital allow you to be able to appreciate the assets that you have and recognise threats that might reduce these?
>
> Finally, compare the format and methodology in the report offered above with that of an assessment published in your locality.

- Public health observatories

> In the UK, public health observatories have been established to provide information for decision making. In the web pages of the Association of Public Health Observatories (APHO)[3] you will find a range of interactive atlases that offer 32 measures to generate your own query. Visit the web page and explore the array of information that can be found by selecting a locality that interests you. The local atlas has six key outcome measure domains, each one housing a cluster of different measures – for example, the indicator 'Adults and health lifestyle' has the following cluster of measures:
>
> Adults who smoke; Binge drinking adults; Healthy eating adults; Physically active adults; Obese adults.
>
> Try comparing the outcomes by running your own query on one of the atlases available on the APHO website www.apho.org.uk/

LETTER 2:   THE SERVICE USER JOURNEY – OUTCOMES

Dear Marie,

Following on from my previous letter about health needs assessment, we know that its purpose is to inform us about service requirements to address identified needs. Once an individual has accessed a service it is necessary to know what its impact has been – whether it was provided as planned and that the quality of provision was upheld. Governance has to maintain service user safety by effective risk management. Beyond this there is also a quest for continual improvement. A recent development in demonstrating service quality is to generate a quality account, which in the United Kingdom is another step in a history of quality reporting stretching back to Florence Nightingale's interest in measurement and categorisation of outcomes into three types: relieved, unrelieved and died.[1]

High Quality Care for All (2008) introduces quality accounts as a mechanism for public reporting on quality.[2] The DoH defines quality of care as 'clinically effective, personal and safe', and adds that it means 'protecting patient safety by eradicating healthcare acquired infections and avoidable accidents. It is about effectiveness of care, from the clinical procedure the patient receives to their quality of life after treatment.' This narrative continues to flag up the importance of the service user's entire experience and the way in which they are treated, including compassion, dignity and respect. In this case, governance is linked to providing a clean, safe and well-managed environment. Whether the account will generate the intended 'truthful and fair picture of the quality of services provided' depends on the measures adopted and the data quality.

Quality measurement is set within a quality framework based on standards that are also audited by an independent regulator (The Care Quality Commission) for the purposes of quality performance management and registration. Its purpose is to 'support improvement with a focus on innovation in medical advances and service design.' Measurement will allow publication of publicly available quality information (as a quality account). Interestingly, this recent (2009) framework notes how quality needs to be *as important to NHS chief executives as it has always been for NHS staff*[3] implying that hitherto it has not been the case.

Standards are necessary to actually measure performance against. These must be SMART – specific, measurable, achievable, realistic and timely. The standard example *'we provide information for prospective service users'* will have a series of SMART statements that an auditor could check to verify that the evidence proves compliance with the standard. Standard setting is a valuable activity as it establishes what should happen and where evidence of compliance should be found.

If you consider the linearity of the service user's journey, each stage of that trajectory can be identified and standards devised to establish what should happen at each point. An example is a preadmission standard where a potential service user is provided with information about a service to facilitate their decision making. The relevant standard might specify that an information pack is provided, perhaps a booklet, perhaps in different languages and containing specific information items. Compliance would be measured by auditing if the standard statements were being met and the evidence to make that assessment could be drawn from qualitative or quantitative sources.

This process is well established, for example, the former Healthcare Commission (now merged into the Care Quality Commission) published its list of ratings – the following example being one about waiting time measures in accident and emergency (A&E). It specifically dealt with the 'measurement of patients waiting less than 12 hours for admission via A&E as an emergency following the decision to admit.' The standard was set along with its rationale that '12 hour waits post decision to admit have been a key target since 2000/01. They remain a marker of unacceptable patient experience'.[4] A rationale is always useful to give auditors a context about the relevance of the measure.

Well Marie, when the service user journey ends, we need to know how well the service performed. That requires measures, and measures require standards.

Yours truly,
Cartmel

Coffee break: knowing what to measure

In this coffee break examine the contemporary policy context of quality accounts, then progress to review notes on how to set standards.

Quality account

For further reading on the details of development of the quality account and how it links to the Care Quality Commission visit the webpage: Department of Health Quality Accounts.[1]

Standards

If you become involved in devising and writing standards there are a series of questions that you need to be aware of based on the SMART acronym.

Specific standards require asking "W" questions:
who is involved; what is required to be achieved; what location; when (time frame) and why?

Measurable standards clearly need criteria for measuring progress towards goal attainment. This keeps the focus on evidence of compliance specific. To know if your goal is measurable ask about quantitative evidence (How much? How many?) and destination – (How will I know when this is achieved?)

Attainable means that the standard has to be achievable. Simply ask yourself: can this be attained; what steps can be taken to ensure that it is attained; in which case, what evidence would you need in order to know when it has been attained?

Realistic standards have an objective that participants are willing and able to work towards achieving. If it is beyond reach it will never be attainable. So what conditions would have to exist to accomplish this goal?

Timely standards have to be achieved within a specified time – A goal should be set within a given time frame. Without this there is no sense of urgency. If you want to lose 10 lb, when do you want to lose it by? "Someday" will not work but if you fit it within a time frame, 'by May 1st', then you have set a destination and date by which you will know one way or the other that you have arrived.

So much for quality frameworks and standards – The question is, do we measure what already exists or do we establish the service we require and then set up measures? The preferable route is the latter – to evaluate the service user journey and develop standards around it.

Decision making: where is it all heading? strategic management

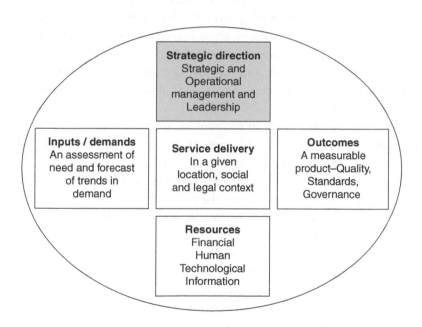

LETTER 1:   STRATEGY: LOST AND FOUND

Dear Marie,

A recent newspaper article ran a story about some people who went trekking in a wilderness area and spent days trying to find their way out of it. That is nothing new – there are some limestone caves near Maastricht in the Netherlands reputed to be a warren that meanders for miles underground and into which people have entered never to find their way out. What can we glean from this? Namely, that people can become so occupied and engrossed with their immediate surroundings that they stop seeing beyond it and run the risk of losing their way. Healthcare managers can also lose their way through deflecting their gaze away from the strategic aims of the organisation. This is why an executive role is necessary to ensure subsidiary functions all work together to achieve the goals of the strategic plan.

Organisational change should not be fragmented – rather it should harmonise with the overall strategic plan and consequently be directly informed by strategic analysis. A strategy is underpinned by values (that you will recall directs behaviour) and translates into achieving goals in designated theme areas. These might be to enhance the research profile, develop evidence-based practice or develop regional expertise. Goals within these themes are achieved in turn through strategic enablers – factors integral to movement towards strategic goals, such as financial stability, valuing and developing staff, and improving effectiveness. In this way, all local actions are developed in the context of a strategic plan reflecting the contribution of the executive strategic function.

In terms of our service model the executive function is to oversee the internal operations as well as to evaluate and assess the external opportunities and threats in order to determine their impact on service continuity and development. To perform these roles strategic skills are necessarily grounded in critical thinking. This is a purposive approach to questioning the external world so as to generate information from which options are identified for the future direction of the organisation. As we know, information relies on data, and that is generated through asking specific questions about the service. So which questions need to be asked about service operations? Have you ever had the experience of not knowing what to ask? This problem can be addressed by categorising features of the external environment so as to be able to focus on specific areas. The subsequent array of questions arising from this methodical examination constitutes the foundation of a minimum data set. The types and modes of data capture can be specified and the database established. The convenience of a database is that it can be used to generate real-time snapshot reports of service operations. These can be represented visually as a 'dashboard' permitting trends to be monitored and emerging risk areas highlighted for intervention. Data management and interpretation are strategic skills necessitating a robust infrastructure to support data capture, recording and processing.

The principle of strategic thinking is evident in accounts of military campaigns. Whilst in some ways these may seem detached from healthcare, they have much to offer in terms of decision making, especially in military autobiographies. These illuminating accounts, when approached with the specific purpose of identifying individual values, focus, information seeking and interpretation provide valuable case studies of the ways in which multiple factors are processed and interpreted to support decision making. The beauty of studying history is that the decision outcomes usually have published competing evaluations so you too can join the fray and think through how you would have performed in that particular set of circumstances.

Professional studies are similarly enhanced through learning from practice. Typically, in a health service we encounter near miss and incident reports that include not only a report of what happened but also an analysis of what contributed to it happening. A root cause analysis is undertaken to recognise contributing factors, and learning and associated actions follow so that the risk of it reoccurring is minimised. When taken collectively across an organisation, common areas of weakness and concern can be identified, and priorities of action determined.

Strategic thinking also encompasses developing a learning culture so that the organisation can record and remember events that have occurred, and to take positive steps to strengthen systems and target staff interventions (education and training) when and where necessary. A strategic-thinking skill set thus requires knowing the current state of the organisation (aided by a minimum data set) as well as reading internal and external environments in order to identify and analyse gaps, and to develop an account of the 'shape' of the future of the organisation. Annual plans will add definition to that shape (as it almost certainly will evolve) and will translate into short- and medium-term achievable goals.

Well Marie, strategic thinking is purposeful and maintains a big picture focus so that the organisation does not lose its way. Having said that some organisations do enter a state of drift – especially family businesses that fail to make effective succession planning. Have you encountered short-term reactive management actions and if so what does that say about strategic thinking?

Yours truly,
Cartmel

Coffee break: not losing the way – strategic function

Strategic function is necessary but might not be highly visible. Workers in some companies have explicit messages articulating the strategic situation to help them to work together and strive to achieve strategic goals. Not all companies are the same, and workers have different levels of investment and engagement with the big picture. Casual staff might be a case in point, perhaps being more occupied with the specific task that they have been engaged to undertake. As part of your reflection on the strategic function in your organisation examine the role of the strategic board. Details of what they do can be found in the following document.

Department of Health (2003): Appointments commission governing the NHS. A guide for NHS Boards.[1]

- Examine it and consider how visible this is within your organisation. What concerns do staff and service users have in your area of work, and where does the strategic function figure in the accounts of these concerns?

The NHS is subject to continuing internal reform and successive waves of political intervention. The King's Fund publication 'Governing the NHS Alternatives to an independent board'[2] provides a critique of how the NHS is governed and offers recommendations to secure a better balance between public accountability, local autonomy and a more devolved healthcare system.

Letter 2:   Where next?

Dear Marie,

Your comments on having read about family businesses that have lost their way through a lack of succession planning and allowing a gap to develop between market requirements and provision is relevant to strategic thinking. I suppose that family businesses illustrate the potency of central controls and reveal the tension encountered when devolving these. When referring to the service model, devolution will always require decisions about where the line is drawn between local autonomy and central control, and this has implications for a unified approach to achieve strategic goals.

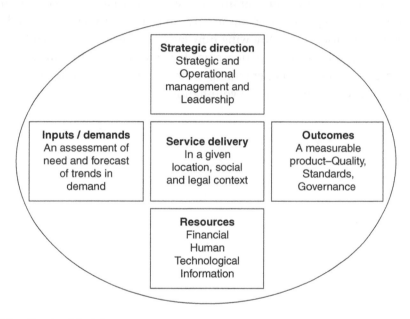

FIGURE 7 Service Model

So let's close our exploration of decision making around service management. The service model can help maintain a focus on provision that has the service user at its heart. Relevant management skills rely on critical thinking about the nature of each element in the model to understand the 'what' or description of each one. Analysis leads you into explanations of why each element exists and how it functions. This leads into questioning of why this is so, and thus opens exploration of what could be different. Your decision making thus falls into two domains – one overseeing the effective and efficient functioning of existing processes, and another that critiques 'what is' in order to consider 'what could be.' The latter type of decision making moves you on from operational management into a strategic arena. You can exercise strategic thinking at a unit level and translate this into service development, especially when sanctioned through devolved authority and accountability. Even if it isn't, there is still scope to lobby for bottom up change, but any progress achieved might be slower.

Management decision making is also about processes and people. Both aspects have their challenges, but effective people management skills will tip the balance between success and frustration in service development.

Well Marie, you have grown as a manager and have honed your critical thinking skills through reflecting on your role over the past months. Decision making lies at the heart of your work – actions arise from decisions, deliberative or intuitive, and this draws on a range of evidence. The service model helps you to identify where this evidence lies – in processes, function and performance, for example. So where do we go from here? You can examine and evaluate your own decision-making expertise as being at a point on a continuum somewhere between novice and expert manager as a decision-maker. Knowing how far you have progressed will be useful in identifying knowledge and experience needed by you to develop further in different management roles – be it operational, strategic or troubleshooting roles. 'Where next?' places the decision making in your hands.

Yours truly,
Cartmel

Decision making in health service management

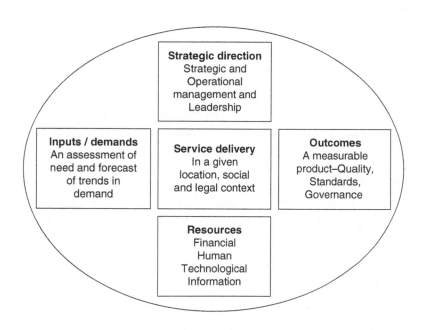

The following module description and learning units are offered as a possible way of using the text as a basis for developing decision-making thinking about service management. The module could be adopted in its entirety or alternatively be selectively used to form learning units that are embedded in other programmes of study.

MODULE DESCRIPTION

Module title   Decision making in health service management

Module aims

The aims of this module are to:

Conceptualise and understand the context of service manager decision making.

Identify roles and skills that service managers possess.

Critically consider the different elements of a service model from a manager's perspective.

Develop an insight into implications of local decision making.

Module content

The module comprises six learning units. Each one focuses on an aspect of real world decision making, linking examination of published evidence and policy to the student's own area of practice.

Learning unit 1: Decision making and the big picture: Making sense of health service delivery

Learning unit 2: Decision making at the heart of service delivery: You as manager?

Learning unit 3: Decision making at the point of service delivery

Learning unit 4: Decision making and resource management

Learning unit 5: Decision making and the service user journey

Learning unit 6: Decision making: Where is it all heading? Strategic management

Skill development

The development of a range of skills forms part of the module activities, including developing communication skills (group discussion and learning feedback), IT (literature searching), problem solving (discussing solutions to service management challenges) and managing personal learning (planning what to study and using resources effectively). These will support professional practice and participation in a range of clinical healthcare management activities.

Teaching and learning strategy

The module can be delivered using a range of learning and teaching strategies designed to meet the learning outcomes. This can include contact teaching sessions, blended learning (e.g. using web-based materials), including supplementary reading to extend learning, classroom or online group work discussion and reflection in order to facilitate individual analysis and learning about current health service management decision making and offer opportunities to develop management decision making competencies in the future.

Students will keep a reflective diary that is structured around the six learning units (corresponding to chapters in the text) to focus on how learning can translate into practical skill development as part of a personal and professional development plan. The coffee break questions could form the basis of weekly online discussion room activities.

Learning outcomes

On successful completion of this module a student will be able to:

1. Explain the context of healthcare service decision making.

2. Understand and explain the elements of a model of service design in relation to their involvement in management decision making.

3. Analyse the care delivery processes in their immediate workplace.

4. Analyse resource management requirements in relation to local service delivery.

5. Understand the service user journey in terms of needs assessment and outcomes.

6. Understand the role of strategic management in service delivery decision making.

ASSESSMENT OF LEARNING
Assignment

The assignment options offer students the opportunity to examine and analyse real world management decision making in their own practice.

The assignment can be adapted to different levels of academic assessment through substitution of different terms in the guidance given (e.g. describe, synthesise, analyse, critically analyse).

Module Pass Requirements

The completion of the assignment to the agreed minimum threshold mark for a pass.

The weighting of the assignment is 100%.

SUGGESTED ASSIGNMENT: AN ANALYSIS OF A MANAGER'S ROLE IN LOCAL SERVICE DELIVERY

A literature study of management decision making in a chosen area of practice
Guidance

Students are to select a chosen area of clinical practice and identify a manager's role within service delivery. This could be the student's own role. They need to provide a brief rationale for this choice and a description of the manager's role.

Option 1 Analysis of a manager's service delivery decision

Identify a decision that the manager makes in service delivery and analyse it in relation to each element of the model provided in the text. The discussion needs to include details on the process of decision making used, including factors that have informed and influenced it. It also needs to include an evaluation of the decision in relation to its intended outcome and identified factors. The concluding section needs to include a discussion about the extent to which an individual manager's decision making can make a difference in service delivery in terms of enabling and inhibiting factors.

Option 2 A literature review of a manager's decision

Undertake a literature review on manager decision making in connection with an identified area of service delivery. The examination of the results needs to be structured around a conceptual framework that draws on the model provided in this text. Using this, the assignment should explain (a) the scope of manager decisions as reported in existing literature (in a chosen area), and (b) identify factors shaping the manager's decisions and (c) the skills thought to be needed by managers in the chosen area. The discussion and conclusion needs to identify a manager skill set, and include a critical discussion of the extent to which practise of these skills would affect service delivery.

Weighting: 100%
Word limit: 3 000

Suggested format of the assignment

1 Title
2 Introduction
3 Search strategy and summary of results
4 A conceptual framework
5 Discussion of the different domains of the conceptual framework
   To include:
   - decision-making definitions
   - theoretical explanations of decision making in the chosen area
   - decision-making context
   - explanations of managers as decision-makers in this area
   - the scope of manager decision making in this chosen area
   - factors shaping decisions
   - skills required of managers as decision-makers
6 Conclusion
   A critical discussion of the extent to which practise of the identified skills would affect service delivery
7 References

How to use the learning units

The six learning units focus on the material in each section of the book. It is recommended that a reflective diary or online discussion board is used to develop personal and shared learning based on the coffee break exercises found at the end of each letter. The reflective diary has two key purposes:

1 To be a live learning tool for students to record their reflections and responses to the coffee break questions.
2 To identify a personal management skill and experience set so that evidence can be produced about existing experience and skills, and to identify and plan how to develop these as well as to acquire new skills.

The letters form the prerequisite reading for each learning unit so that classroom-based learning can concentrate group exploration of particular issues. The coffee break exercises often contain links to additional resources so as to offer an opportunity for students to extend the scope of their learning about a given topic.

LEARNING UNITS

1 DECISION MAKING AND THE BIG PICTURE – MAKING SENSE OF HEALTH SERVICE DELIVERY

The aims of learning unit 1 are:
Examine representations of organisational design.
Examine a model of organisational design.
Examine mission, vision and purpose.
Examine stakeholders and stakeholder focus.
Examine the meaning of the term 'health'.

Text reference – Section 1
Learning outcomes – 1

Learning content	Staff contribution	Student exercises	Learning resources
1 Organisational design	Introduce the real world of the experience of front-line service delivery using a case study as an illustration. Lead a discussion about what components are required to deliver a service.	Group discussion about the different components that are required to provide a service.	Letter 1
2 Examine a model of organisational design	Present the model and build it up element by element.	Reflect on and discuss the extent to which the model explains the student's experience of healthcare service delivery.	Letter 2
3 Examine mission, vision and purpose	Discuss the definitions of mission, vision and purpose. Use real examples to demonstrate how these are expressed and differ across different organisations. Lead a group analysis to determine what is the same, what differs and why there might be differences, as well as to consider the underpinning values within the service.	Identify different expressions of mission, vision and purpose. Review the value base behind mission, vision and purpose statements. Discuss the implications of different values operating within subgroups of the organisation.	Letters 3 and 4. Examples of healthcare provider mission, vision and purpose statements.

Learning content	Staff contribution	Student exercises	Learning resources
4 Examine stakeholders and stakeholder interest	Lead group identification of internal and external stakeholders using the model. Discuss internal and external threats to the organisation's focus, and also whether this focus should remain stable or be open to change.	Identify stakeholders associated with each element of the model. Identify external stakeholders. Review which are the most powerful in terms of shaping the mission, vision and purpose of the organisation. Discuss how weaker stakeholders could increase their influence on the organisation.	Letters 5 and 6. Use the model as a tool to label different stakeholders.
5 Examine the meaning of the term 'health'	Continuing with the focus on the organisation, examine definitions of health and the extent to which particular ones are evident in the statements of mission, vision and purpose.	Review definitions of health and evaluate the implications for the type of service provided according to which definition is adopted.	Letter 7
6 Summary	Revisit the overview of organisational design, mission vision and purpose, and how stakeholders shape this, even to the extent of bringing into scrutiny competing views of how health is understood within the service.	Students are directed to identify the meaning of health within their own workplace.	Refer to the coffee break points.

Learning unit summary

By the end of this learning unit students will have examined representations of health service organisations, and used the model as a tool to offer structure to thinking how we might think about healthcare organisations and decision making within them. This will have included identifying factors that shape expressions of the organisation (mission, vision and purpose). Finally, definitions of health will have been considered in relation to stakeholders and the focus of the healthcare organisation.

Reflective diary

The student is asked to maintain a reflective diary based on the coffee break questions linked to each letter. Some of these are included below.

Coffee break: Reference for discussion

1 **Coffee break: organisational design**
Spend some time exploring and reflecting on the design of your local organisation.
   - Examine and describe the organisational design of your local service – what do you think comprises its constituent parts, and how are these arranged and interrelated?
   - How would you represent it as a diagram? (When making sense of complex situations it can help to sketch out different ways in which constituent parts can be represented in relation to each other.)
   - Does the arrangement that you have sketched have a particular shape, and does this have any significance in representing where service delivery decisions are made and how they are supported? Is there an 'official' representation of the shape of your healthcare organisation? If it differs from your initial sketch does this raise any challenges to your account of where service delivery decisions are made and how they are supported?

2 **Coffee break: models, purpose, mission and vision**
Here are some questions to help develop your initial exploration of your local organisation.
   - Use the model as a route map and determine the extent to which it helps to explain the local organisation. What fits? Where does it fit? What else can you add within the elements of the model? Can you see any new elements emerging?
   - What is the explicit purpose of your chosen local healthcare organisation?
   - What, if any, is the published mission and vision?

3 **Coffee break: purpose, mission and vision translated into practice**
Take time to consider how statements of purpose, mission, vision and values translate into the real world practice of service delivery.
   - What leads the workforce to live the values? (Many role descriptions require applicants to support and uphold the organisation's values; others require staff to live their values.)
   - How can an organisation ensure that its values are supported?
   - To what extent do the values of the employing organisation match your values?
   - If values differ do compromises need to be made that cause conflicts of conscience?
   - In what ways does labelling a service user as a patient or customer reflect the perspective of the organisation?

4 **Coffee break: promoting ownership**
Take time to explore ways in which ownership is achieved in your local workplace.
   - Look around your local unit and reflect on what you hear and observe regarding vision, and ask 'does this promote ownership or not?'
   - What methods are used to communicate and translate vision into practice?
   - Vision and ownership – to what extent does being 'off message' challenge the local organisation?
   - What organisational response does being 'off message' generate?
   - When can being 'off message' be healthy?
   - What does an organisation lose when it seeks to shed staff who previously worked under a different executive and vision?

5 **Coffee break: identifying stakeholders**

Consider the organisational model and each of its elements to determine who the stakeholders are.

- Who are the stakeholders within each element?
- Who are the stakeholders outside of the organisation?
- Are some stakeholders more influential than others? If so, why?

6 **Coffee break: decisions and stakeholders**

You will be making service delivery decisions that are linked to each area of the organisation depicted in the model. These decisions will acknowledge stakeholder involvement and be bounded in certain ways.

- Revisit your description of the decision-making process in relation to stakeholder involvement. A diagram might help to clarify the steps in the decision making process.
- What role and information might each identified stakeholder contribute to your decision making?
- How can you access the information that each stakeholder provides?
- What types of decisions do the stakeholders make? How might this be useful to know when making service delivery decisions?

7 **Coffee break: interpreting the meaning of health**

There are different interpretations of health. Whichever is adopted will directly shape service purpose and design. It will also inform the design of measures to evaluate whether or not health interventions have been effective. So what is the dominant interpretation of health in your local service?

- Locate an explicit account of how the organisation expresses and therefore interprets the meaning of health.
- Do different interpretations exist within different parts of the organisation?
- If so, how do these find expression, and what are the implications for service design and delivery?

2 DECISION MAKING AT THE HEART OF SERVICE DELIVERY: YOU AS MANAGER?

The aims of learning unit 2 are:
To examine the role and tasks undertaken by health service managers.
To explore how understanding people is central to managing services.
To examine whether managers can 'hit the ground running' before understanding the local context.
To examine the internal and external environment of a service in relation to decision making.

Text reference – Section 2
Learning outcomes – 1,2,3

Learning content	Staff contribution	Student exercises	Learning resources
1 Introduction: What do healthcare managers do?	Link to the previous learning unit and move on to focus on the manager's role. Lead the group to synthesise and recount the different roles of a manager and tasks that they perform in service delivery.	Group exercise (e.g. on a white board or flip chart) to list and categorise the scope and details of management role and tasks in frontline service delivery. Begin to identify the competencies that are linked to each task.	Letter 1
2 How do managers manage?	Having identified tasks and roles, lead discussion on examples of open and closed management styles. Include in the discussion the effects of these on the way teams work.	Consider the impact of different management styles on staff teams. Continue to identify behavioural traits that foster good teamwork and team contribution.	Letter 2
3 Hit the ground running?	Introduce the idea of bringing an outside manager into a service to take charge of it and develop it. Explore the extent to which this is feasible.	Discuss whether it is possible to move a service forward without investing time to understand the local organisation and work culture. What would be the advantages and disadvantages of this approach to achieving effective change?	Letter 3

Learning content	Staff contribution	Student exercises	Learning resources
4 Decision making and change: Reading the environment	Take an example of a service delivery decision in one of the student's workplaces and facilitate the group to analyse the factors shaping that decision within the workplace and outside of it. Lead the students to develop a description of their decision-making process to identify logical points where different factors shape the overall process of decision making.	Identify factors shaping a service delivery decision to recognise the complexity of the situation. Discuss which factors are controllable and which are not. What is the implication of both of them on service decisions.	Letter 4
5 Summary	Conclude the learning unit with a review of the different roles and tasks undertaken by different health service managers, drawing out similarities and differences between them.		Refer to the coffee break points.

Learning unit summary

By the end of this learning unit students will have examined what service delivery managers do as well as aspects of role tasks, associated competencies and also their relationship with other staff in the workplace. The merits of promoting change by introducing new managers into the workplace will have been reviewed. Finally, a real world decision will have been used as an illustration to identify factors shaping service delivery.

Reflective diary

The student is asked to maintain a reflective diary based on the coffee break questions linked to each letter. Some of these are included below.

1 **Coffee break: what are your management roles and competencies?**
Which management role competencies do you need?
Next read the key skills framework to identify some competencies linked to the roles that you have identified.
How big is the task?
Using the summary provided in section 2 (from the NHS graduate scheme) read it in the context of the model provided to see where the narrative corresponds to its elements, and consider what is 'best management' and which competency set would match this.

2 **Coffee break: understanding people to manage people**
The skill of understanding human nature and reading behaviour lies at the heart of management. It is not enough to be a manager who is technically excellent regarding systems and process having a portfolio of task competencies but lacks essential 'people skills.' This reflection is really an ongoing issue to keep revisiting. It is about understanding people and working with them.
- Which information sources do you access to learn about people, their nature and behaviour?
- What is the nature of person?
- What do you base your perspective on?
- How sufficient is this perspective?
- What is the implication of your perspective in terms of translating it into actions based on truthfulness, collaboration, fairness, transparency, advocacy and firmness?
- How do you manage situations where there is a diversity of perspectives about the nature of person?

3 **Coffee break: role continuity or change?**
If you had a skills deficit in a team you could employ the right person to fit the requirement – the round peg for the round hole. Thatis useful and can happen in cases where short-term relief cover is required (such as a 6 month maternity leave of absence). Consider what additional value might be added to the practice of managing others by accepting that a post is more than 'a peg in a hole' and that the 'hole' might need to be refashioned, and so the 'peg' altered to match the new requirement.
- Can you detect any assumptions about how the local organisation understands the role of the manager?
- What indications are there that this is up for negotiation by post-holders?
- What is the process by which this might be achieved?
- How would a change in the manager's role impact on other aspects of the model?
- In cases where the scope of the manager's role is not negotiable what is the organisation likely to lose and gain?

4 **Coffee break: reading the environment**
Use this break to do two tasks –
1 Identify current changes in the external environment (use a PEST framework: political, economic, social, technological dimensions) and use the guide below to think through what the implications for local actions might be.
Use this guide -
- Read the external and internal environments
- Assess the impact this will have
- Generate decision options
- Act

Then look through your local major incident plan to see the scope of events included and procedures for responding to them.

2 To add to the scope of your knowledge about major incident planning check out relevant online guidance, beginning with the resources offered below. You will find more examples of healthcare disaster plans in the public domain.

- Planning for the evacuation and sheltering of people in health sector settings: interim strategic national guidance.[1]
- Examples of good practice in emergency planning.[2]
- You might consider how thinking about safe process design can provide a robust approach to planning – The Health and Safety Executive have advice available to refer to.[3]

3 DECISION MAKING AT THE POINT OF SERVICE DELIVERY

The aims of learning unit 3 are:
Examine and explain governance and risk reporting.
Examine and explore governance and smart working processes.
Examine governance and workforce development.

Text reference – Section 3
Learning outcomes – 3, 4 and 5

	Learning content	Staff contribution	Student exercises	Learning resources
1	Introduction: Governance and risk reporting	Link to the previous learning unit, and focus on governance and safe systems of work. Draw out using real world examples like failures in service delivery that highlight deficient governance.	Discuss how governance and risk reporting is undertaken in the workplace. What promotes an open culture for risk reporting?	Letter 1
2	Governance and smart working processes	Discuss the difference between incremental development of a service and a transformational development. Discuss how a business plan can help to clarify thinking about service development.	Identify and discuss some barriers to effective and efficient working.	Letter 2
3	Governance and workforce development	Returning to a theme in an earlier learning unit, revisit the value of the workforce in relation to service development and delivery.	Examine and describe the intellectual capital in the students' own workplaces – how is this understood and anticipate the effect of eroding that resource.	Letter 3
4	Summary	Draw together the key points about governance and safe systems. Then highlight the centrality of the workforce in ensuring governance works. Finally highlight the risk to effective governance when intellectual capital is lost through staff leaving.employment.		Refer to the coffee break points.

Learning unit summary

By the end of this learning unit students will have examined clinical governance, efficient and effective ways of working, and the place of a business plan in focusing on how to effect change. The intellectual capital of the workforce will have been explored in relation to maintaining effective governance.

Reflective log

The student is asked to maintain a reflective log based on the coffee break questions linked to each letter. Some of these are included below.

---

1   **Coffee break: managing processes: governance and risk reporting**
1 Risk

In letter 1 (section 2) it was noted that you could work out which systems of care delivery are needed by referring to the relevant legislation and regulatory requirements. A summary of regulations relevant to the workplace is provided by the HSE (2008). Employers are required to carry out risk assessments, make arrangements to implement necessary measures and appoint competent people as well as to arrange for appropriate information and training.

Select one example from these and examine the detail of what is included so that you can:

* Understand how risk assessments related to these are undertaken in your workplace.
* Identify the measures to address the risks.
* What training and information is provided in relation to those measures?
* Finally, how has this regulation been applied to yourself during your employment?

2 Reporting of injuries, diseases and dangerous occurrences regulations

Certain accidents and diseases have to be reported under the Reporting of Injuries, Diseases and Dangerous Occurrences Regulations (1995). 'Reporting accidents and ill health at work is a legal requirement. The information enables the Health and Safety Executive (HSE) and Local Authorities, to identify where and how risks arise, and to investigate serious accidents'.[1]

Look through the RIDDOR web pages (or equivalent if you are working in a different country) to know the criteria for making a report and how you would do this. These include deaths, major injuries, specific minor injuries and dangerous occurrences (near misses). For specific details see the web page.[2]

3 Health and safety

The Health and Safety at Work Act 1974[3] explicitly outlines employer and employee responsibilities in the workplace. Ownership of these responsibilities by staff will happen when they understand safe working practices and how these can become part of everyday practice, hence the need for training. Look at the heath and safety executive website to review the Act which is primary legislation, and secondary Acts called Statutory Instruments. I want you to specifically read the enforcement section within the website and look through examples from the following three different types of enforcement – prosecutions, improvement notices and prohibition notices so that you gain an appreciation of what can happen and the fines imposed if this aspect of providing a safe working environment is neglected.

2 **Coffee break: governance, smart working processes and the business plan**

Having considered the patient journey and the configuration of services around it, consider lean thinking and ways of reducing waste and plan to improve services, and robust governance.

1 Lean thinking

Map out the service user journey for your service.

Identify the participants, processes and resources associated with that journey.

Adopting a 'Lean Thinking' approach and identify examples of types of waste in the journey.

Having identified some areas of waste think how they could be addressed and translated into action steps of change?

2 Business plans to translate ideas into practice

Having identified process development needs you need to think about how all the participants will 'buy into' the proposed change. One method is to specify the details of this change in a business plan. The format for a business case is a variation on a theme and might have a particular house style but should include the following:

- An executive summary
- A short description of the business opportunity
- People involved
- Your communications and implementation plans
- Your management team and personnel
- Your operations
- Financial forecasts

Thus, a business plan might be a way of formalising planned change into an achievable and resourced trajectory. Finally, spend some time exploring clinical governance as a method of implementing systems management within a healthcare organisation.

3 Clinical governance

<u>Why clinical governance?</u> Why do you think that we need clinical governance models and what predated these in clinical services? Why did former health service arrangements need to change in the UK? A way to understand this can be found in the historical account included in Palmer's (2002) article.[1]

<u>A definition of clinical governance</u>. Quality services arrayed around the patient journey require governing to ensure that harmony and synergies serve the chief purpose. Clinical governance is the system through which organisations 'are accountable for continuously improving the quality of their services and safeguarding high standards of care, by creating an environment in which clinical excellence will flourish'.[2]

The Royal College of Nursing described it as 'the mechanism by which the public can be assured that NHS organisations have comprehensive and robust systems in place for continuously improving the quality of their services and safeguarding high standards of clinical care. It is the framework through which all the components of quality, including patient and public involvement, are brought together and placed high on the agenda of each organisation'.[3]

Representing clinical governance. One means of representing this is the seven pillars of clinical governance model developed by the NHS Clinical Governance Support team. In this model the apex of governance is partnership between the patient and the professional in decisions about treatment and care. The seven pillars are clinical effectiveness, clinical audit, risk management, patient experience, communication, resource management and learning. A different version of a governance model can be found in an Australian publication at www. safetyandquality.health.wa.gov.au (Refer to section 2 for reference details.)

3 **Coffee break: intellectual and social capital**
1 Recognising change

When you manage staff effectively, their experience of work can be fulfilling and productive, which in turn contributes to workforce stability. This has an impact on service quality. This investment is not to be underestimated, but change can threaten this stability. Indeed, it can be a catalyst that prompts staff to leave employment, which is sometimes euphemistically called 'career development.' Just as the patient has a journey, so do staff. In this coffee break consider the challenges to workforce stability in your workplace.

- Revisit the staff journey from initial interest in a post through to their leaving employment.
- What is the rate of staff turnover in your unit over the past year?
- How does this compare to the whole organisation over the same period?
- What changes are impacting on your workplace?
- How is this impacting on the local workforce?
- Draw a force field diagram to analyse factors supporting and resisting change in your workplace. Which factors could be controlled to promote staff retention (workforce stability)? Which factors cannot be controlled and what are the implications of these for you as a manager?
- How does knowing about controllable and uncontrollable factors inform your approach to managing staff and promoting team stability?

2 The impact of staff turnover

When a staff member leaves their post, the unit loses more than just a person who undertook so many hours of work per week. It loses local knowledge, experience and expertise. I call this intellectual capital. Additionally, it loses a part of a social network, a character with an interpersonal skill set, a colleague, even a friend of the staff team – this I call social capital. Whilst no one is indispensable, a team can encounter a sense of loss, and tangibly so when a staff member retires or even dies in post.

- In terms of professional decision making how would you describe the value of the intellectual capital in your unit?
- What effect might the loss of intellectual capital have on professional decision making and patient safety?
- How does loss of social capital weaken the stability of the workforce?
- How do your reflections on intellectual and social capital inform your approach to managing staff?

4 DECISION MAKING AND RESOURCE MANAGEMENT

The aims of learning unit 4 are:
Examine the staff journey – to recognise the investment made in the workforce.
Examine communication and communication channels supporting governance.
Examine health informatics in service delivery.

Text reference – Section 4
Learning outcomes – 3 and 4

	Learning content	Staff contribution	Student exercises	Learning resources
1	Introduction: Governance and the staff journey	Linking to the previous learning unit, pick up on the theme of intellectual capital to direct attention on to the considerable investment made in the workforce.	Take the trajectory of the staff journey and identify the manager's skills needed at each stage so as to be able to develop a related skill set and associated competencies.	Letter 1
2	Managing information and communication	Make the point that communication is often the weak point in service delivery, especially when investigating incidents. Facilitate the group to identify the organisation of information in service delivery and to think about how this can be managed.	Identify the communication channels in the workplace and the types of information as well as the gates and safeguards to information disclosure. What should govern sharing and access to information?	Letter 2
3	Health informatics	Discuss the use of computers in healthcare and the impact that has on working practices in service delivery. What are the gains and losses?	Review the use of computers in the students' workplaces and how that impacts on information access, sharing and security.	Letter 3
4	Summary	Draw the session to a close, by highlighting that people, communication and information systems are key resources integral to service delivery.		Refer to the coffee break points

Learning unit summary

By the end of this learning unit students will have examined decision making and resource management – particularly the investment in the staff journey, communication systems and informatics.

Reflective log

The student is asked to maintain a reflective log based on the coffee break questions linked to each letter. Some of these are included below.

1 **Coffee break: governance and management style**

1 Managing staff – being an encourager

You might have heard the light-hearted saying that 'the beatings will continue until morale improves'. Whilst humorous, it is like the story of a donkey pulling a cart – the driver beats the donkey if it does not move whilst dangling a carrot in front of the donkey to entice it forward. This carrot and stick approach might describe an organisational approach to workforce management – stick by threatened sanctions and carrots through staff development opportunities.

- To what extent can you detect this in your own organisation?
- If this is the case, how could it be altered?
- Do staff need to have boundaries that when crossed trigger sanctions?
- Is it possible to attain a state within a team where the boundary of sanctions is not needed?
- Where do disciplinary rules fit into a carrot and stick analogy?

2 Managing staff – disciplinary action

Managers have to deal with disciplinary matters, and disciplinary procedure is designed to deal with situations where behaviour falls below an acceptable standard. Look up your organisation's disciplinary policy and procedure. Particularly note the different types of disciplinary offence and the levels of response as well as the sanction that is applied.

Compare your local organisation's disciplinary procedure with advice provided on the Chartered Institute of Personnel and Development (CIPD) website 'The HR and development website'.[1] Next compare your local organisation's guidance with that provided by the advisory, conciliation and arbitration service (ACAS). ACAS provides information on grievance procedures and the disciplinary process. ACAS's purpose is stated as: 'We aim to improve organisations and working life through better employment relations. We help with employment relations by supplying up-to-date information, independent advice and high quality training, and working with employers and employees to solve problems and improve performance.'[2]

Look at the following examples of disciplinary action, and having studied them, how do these inform your vigilance as a manager to recognise breaches of discipline? What can you do to develop your vigilance to protect the integrity of the service?

Hospital sacks senior manager over stolen laptop

- Health chiefs in Colchester fired a senior manager who lost confidential records on thousands of patients after his hospital laptop was stolen[3]

Press release: Police in hospital deaths inquiry[4]

- Nurse dismissed after four patients die in intensive care unit

Case studies of recent NHS fraud cases[5]

- Timesheet fraud, stealing drugs, forgery, failing to carry out safety checks

3 Managing staff – which style?

If effective management of the organisation's most valuable asset is essential, what approach will you take? In many management texts you will read about democratic, autocratic, consultative and laissez-faire management styles. Your management style may lead to greater motivation and productivity from your staff. However, it is not as simple as just 'picking' a style as individual personalities and characteristics influence this. Read the following summaries and consider the extent to which any of these describe your style. Can your management style alter according to the situation? If so, what factors shape your choice of a different style? Does staff prefer a particular management style – or is it impossible to generalise?

Democratic management style

A democratic manager delegates authority to their staff so that they take the responsibility to complete the task given to them. Staff will complete their tasks using their own work methods; Through including staff in decision making it engenders ownership and enhances motivation, which has an impact on the quality of decision making and work outcomes. On the other hand a democratic management style can actually slow decision making due to the need for consultation.

Autocratic management style

An autocratic manager dictates orders to their staff and makes decisions without any consultation. They prefer control and quick decisions so that work is usually completed on time. However, because of this approach staff motivation can decrease and staff turnover increases.

Consultative management style

A consultative style is a combination of the above two. The manager will ask for views and opinions from their staff, allowing them to feel involved, but will ultimately make the final decision.

Laissez-faire management style

A laissez-faire manager sets the tasks and gives staff complete freedom to complete the task as they see fit with minimal involvement. The manager acts as a coach and provides information if required. It has the benefit of staff ownership and development, and may lead to improved motivation. Its drawback can be that with little direction staff may feel lost and not reach their goals.

2 **Coffee break: freedom of information and communications strategy**
In this coffee break begin by looking through the Freedom of Information Act (FOIA): that is accessible via the information commissioner's office (ICO)[1] and consider the following:
When is information 'caught' by the FOIA?
What is the duty to confirm or deny the existence of information?
What is exempted from the FOIA?
What is the Public Interest test? Refer to the Freedom of Information Act Awareness Guidance No 3 The Public Interest Test 1. March 2007 ICO.
Look through the list of absolute and qualified exemptions in the Act.

Whilst the FOIA deals with specifics regarding decisions about disclosure, a broader debate surrounds the place of the dividing line between the disclosure and withholding information.

In terms of external communications what should the public know and not know about a service and its performance?
How would a senior manager decide what the public should be told?

What process does your local organisation stipulate that should be followed when making a disclosure?

Are there advantages to keeping information from the public?

Why could it be beneficial?

What problems are caused by withholding information from the public?

What criteria should be used to make decisions about disclosure?

Now turn your study to familiarising yourself with examples of communication strategies. Undertake a simple web search (try typing: 'NHS Trust Communication strategy' into a search engine) and examine the aims and objectives of the strategies to note the commonality amongst them.

Here are two to get you started:

These particular examples illustrate the aims and objectives of a robust communications strategy.

1 The aims are about communicating and sharing the values of the organisation, engendering the publics' trust in the service and communicating the strategic direction.[2]

2 Typically, statements of aims will read 'To help the Trust to successfully communicate both internally and externally, thereby contributing to the achievement of its aims and objectives'.[3]

3 **Coffee break: local procedures and information management**

Take time to examine local information management procedures specifically focusing on the following:

Data Protection Act

Data security

Passwords and patient identifiable data

Contemporary communication – what do you think?

I was at an exhibition recently at the War Museum North about 'Animals at war.' Prominent in one of the display cases was a stuffed pigeon and photographic illustrations of how these had message canisters attached to them. Aeroplane crews would release them during operations over enemy territory so that secure messages could be sent back to base. That was quite an ingenious yet simple formal communication system that proved to be functional. Other communication channels have included lamps (to send line of sight messages as a series of Morse code dots and dashes), radio, telephone and publications. Contemporary developments have included podcasts, blogs, wikis and networking sites (face book). The point is that there are different ways of formally communicating information either visually, verbally or in objects such as written text (by formal I mean in a planned and approved way). Access to such communication will include granting permission to access the information, and providing the skills and equipment needed to receive and use it. – even using a telephone is a skill to be learnt, just as was caring for a carrier pigeon.

What is your definition of effective communication?

What is your definition of efficient communication?

What steps can be taken to support effective electronic communication within your workplace?

What are the enablers and barriers to supporting effective electronic communication in the workplace?

How might you minimise these barriers?

How will a paperless office enhance or impede your work?

5 DECISION MAKING AND THE SERVICE USER JOURNEY

The aims of learning unit 5 are:
Examine and understand the service user journey from the perspective of manager decision making.
Understand how services can be measured and how decisions about measurements are made.

Text reference – Section 5
Learning outcomes – 3 and 5

	Learning content	Staff contribution	Student exercises	Learning resources
1	Introduction: Health needs assessment	Having examined resource management, attention is now turned to two ends of the service user journey – health needs assessment and outcomes.	Discuss how health needs can be assessed and how needs can be measured. How does the method of assessment shape the design of services?	Letter 1
2	The service user journey: Outcomes	Lead discussion on how service outcomes should be measured? What should be measured and is measurement the only way of evaluating outcomes?	Identify what can be measured and what is difficult to measure. What are the political implications of outcome measurement? To what extent is outcome measurement a reflection of the team or other factors?	Letter 2
3	Summary	Draw together the point that service design and management is bound up with measurement. The stakeholder control of decisions about what is measured shapes the design of services and the understanding of how well it is performing.		Refer to the coffee break points

Learning unit summary
By the end of this learning unit students will have examined ways of knowing patients, the scope and depth of a narrative, the report process and judgements used to summarise how patients are known.

Reflective log
The student is asked to maintain a reflective log based on the coffee break questions linked to each letter. Some of these are included below.

1 **Coffee break: health needs assessment**
This coffee break can be spent reviewing the guidance provided to undertake a health needs assessment and then seeing the detail of real examples. You might need a refill by the time you get to the end of this!

The process of health needs assessment
The process of health needs assessment is provided in more detail in this NICE (NIHCE) publication: Summary: Health needs assessment at a glance.[1]

Read the guide and then inspect a real example of a health needs assessment. There are many that can be easily accessed on the internet – one specific example is Swansea's health social care and well-being (HSCWB) needs assessment (2007).[2]

Note particularly the health map and determinants of health and well-being (page 5). How do these determinants compare with those used in your locality?

Social capital is mentioned in the above report – (page 31). What similarities can you see between this and the social and intellectual capital within the staff group in your service? How does defining social and intellectual capital allow you to be able to appreciate the assets that you have and recognise threats that might reduce these?
Finally, compare the format and methodology in the report offered above with that of an assessment published in your locality.

Public health observatories
In the UK public health observatories have been established to provide information about decision making. In the web pages of the Association of Public Health Observatories (APHO)[3] you will find a range of interactive atlases that offer 32 measures to generate your own query. Visit the web page and explore the array of information that can be found by selecting a locality that interests you. The local atlas has six key outcome measure domains, each one housing a cluster of different measures – for example, the indicator 'adults and health lifestyle' has the following cluster of measures:

Adults who smoke; binge drinking adults; healthy eating adults; physically active adults; obese adults.

Try comparing the outcomes by running your own query on one of the atlases available on the APHO website www.apho.org.uk/

2 **Coffee break: knowing what to measure**
In this coffee break examine the contemporary policy context of quality accounts, then progress to review notes on how to set standards.

Quality account
For further reading on the details of development of the quality account and how it links to the Care Quality Commission visit the following webpage: Department of Health Quality Accounts.[1]

Standards
If you become involved in setting and writing standards there are a series of questions that you need to be aware of based on the SMART acronym.
    Specific standards require asking "W" questions:
    Who is involved; what is required to be achieved; what location; when (time frame) and why?

Measurable standards clearly need criteria for measuring progress towards goal attainment. This keeps the focus on evidence of compliance specific. To know if your goal is measurable ask about quantitative evidence (How much? How many?), and destination – (How will I know when this is achieved?)

Attainable means that the standard has to be achievable. Simply ask yourself: can this be attained; what steps can be taken to ensure that it is attained; in which case, what evidence would you need in order to know when it has been attained?

Realistic standards have an objective that participants are willing and able to work towards achieving. If it is beyond reach it will never be attainable. So what conditions would have to exist to accomplish this goal?

Timely standards have to be achieved within a specified time – A goal should be set within a given time frame. Without this there is no sense of urgency. If you want to lose 10 lb, when do you want to lose it by? "Someday" will not work but if you fit it within a time frame, 'by May 1st', then you have set a destination and date by which you will know one way or the other that you have arrived.

So much for quality frameworks and standards – The question is, do we measure what already exists or do we establish the service we require and then set up measures? The preferable route is the latter – to evaluate the service user journey and develop standards around it.

6 DECISION MAKING: WHERE IS IT ALL HEADING? STRATEGIC MANAGEMENT

The aims of learning unit 6 are:

Examine the strategic function as it applies to local service delivery

Understand that management decision making is concerned with people and processes.

Text reference – Section 6
Learning outcomes – 6

	Learning content	Staff contribution	Student exercises	Learning resources
1	Introduction: Losing the way	This final learning unit draws together the elements of the model and questions why organisations might encounter strategic drift – losing their way. Examples might be used, such as organisations that develop too broad a focus and have to reorganise to reclaim a distinctive focus.	Discuss the explicit strategic vision of a selected healthcare organisation. Examine factors that cause organisations to lose a distinctive focus.	Letter 1
2	Keeping a focus	Decision making lies at the heart of your service delivery management. The service model helps students to identify where in the organization they are located and the decisions that they should make as a result. Lead the students to examine and evaluate their own decision-making expertise (as being at a point on a continuum somewhere between novice and expert manager as a decision-maker). Continue into an evaluation of personal skills inventories – places where manager decision-making expertise and experience already exists and places where it is identified as needing to be developed.	Having understood both the macro and micro aspects of service management, students now review their place in their own workplace organisation – critiquing the clarity of vision and direction, and the personal implication of this as decision-making managers.	Letter 2

Learning content	Staff contribution	Student exercises	Learning resources
3 Summary	The series of learning units have been used to draw out aspects of service management.	Review the personal reflective log to evaluate how understanding of manager roles and tasks have developed over the period of study	

Learning unit summary

By the end of this learning unit students will have examined the strategic function and its relationship to local service delivery. They will also have reviewed management decision making as being about processes and people.

Reflective log

The student is asked to maintain a reflective log based on the coffee break questions linked to each letter. Some of these are included below.

1 **Coffee Break: not losing the way: strategic function**

Strategic function is necessary but might not be highly visible. Workers in some companies have explicit messages articulating the strategic situation to help them to work together and strive to achieve strategic goals. Not all companies are the same, and workers have different levels of investment and engagement with the big picture. Casual staff might be a case in point, perhaps being more occupied with the specific task that they have been engaged to undertake. As part of your reflection on the strategic function in your organisation examine the role of the strategic board. Details of what they do can be found in the following document.

Department of Health (2003): Appointments commission governing the NHS. A guide for NHS Boards.[1] Examine it and consider how visible this is within your organisation. What concerns do staff and service users have in your area of work, and where does the strategic function figure in the accounts of these concerns?

References

SECTION 1 DECISION MAKING AND THE BIG PICTURE: MAKING SENSE OF HEALTH SERVICE DELIVERY

Letter 1: The main focus

Coffee break: organisational design

Letter 2: Representing health service complexity – the big picture

Coffee break: models, purpose, mission and vision

Letter 3: Purpose – mission and vision
1 Lancashire Teaching Hospitals NHS Trust. Annual Plan 2007/2008. Available at: www.lancsteachinghospitals.nhs.uk/media/annual_plan_07-08.pdf (accessed 3 December 2010).
2 Church of England. Holy Communion (Order One). Available at: www.cofe.anglican.org/worship/liturgy/commonworship/texts/hc/orderone.html (accessed 3 December 2010).
3 Lancashire Teaching Hospitals NHS Trust Annual Plan 2007/2008. Available at: www.lancsteachinghospitals.nhs.uk/media/annual_plan_07-08.pdf (accessed 3 December 2010).
4 Guys and St Thomas NHS Trust. Our Values'. Available at: www.guysandstthomas.nhs.uk/about/strategic/ourvalues.aspx (accessed 3 December 2010).
5 Guys and St Thomas NHS Trust Our Values'. Available at: www.guysandstthomas.nhs.uk/about/strategic/ourvalues.aspx (accessed 3 December 2010).
6 St. Mary's Hospital Amsterdam New York. Available at: www.smha.org/ (accessed 3 December 2010).
7 Toronto Mount Sinai Hospital Vision Mission Values. Available at: www.mtsinai.on.ca/AboutUs/Images/VisionMissionValues.pdf (accessed 3 December 2010).

Coffee break: purpose, mission and vision translated into practice

Letter 4: Purpose, mission, vision and ownership

Coffee break: promoting ownership

Letter 5: Shifting focus

Coffee break: identifying stakeholders

Letter 6: Whose service is it? – stakeholders

1 Department of Health. The NHS Improvement Plan 2004. Available at: www.dh.gov. uk/en/Publicationsandstatistics/Publications/PublicationsPolicyAndGuidance/ DH_4084476 (accessed 3 December 2010).
2 Department of Health. NHS in England: The operating framework for 2006/7. Available at: www.dh.gov.uk/en/AdvanceSearchResult/index.htm?searchTerms=operating +framework+2006%2F7 (accessed 3 December 2010).
3 Department of Health. Commission for Patient and Public Involvement in Health. Available at: www.dh.gov.uk/en/Managingyourorganisation/PatientAndPublic involvement/index.htm (accessed 3 December 2010).
4 Department of Health. Patient and Public Involvement Forums. Available at: www.dh.gov.uk/en/Managingyourorganisation/PatientAndPublicinvolvement/ DH_4074577 (accessed 3 December 2010).
5 Department of Health. Local Involvement Networks (LINks). Available at: www.dh.gov.uk/en/Managingyourorganisation/PatientAndPublicinvolvement/ DH_076366 (accessed 3 December 2010).

Coffee break: decisions and stakeholders

Letter 7: The big picture – what is the meaning of health in a health service?

1 Herodotus. *The Histories Book*. London: Penguin; 1;197. pp. 87.
2 Ashdown M. *A Complete System of Nursing*. London: J.M. Dent and Sons; 1943. pp. 3.
3 Talcott Parsons cited in Aggleton, P. 1990 *Health*. London: Routledge; pp. 10.
4 World Health Organization. Constitution of the World Health Organization 1946. Available at: apps.who.int/gb/bd/PDF/bd46/e-bd46_p2.pdf (accessed 3 December 2010).
5 World Health Organization 1981. Global Strategy for Health for all by the year 2000. Available at: whqlibdoc.who.int/publications/9241800038.pdf (accessed 3 December 2010).

Coffee break: interpreting the meaning of health

SECTION 2 DECISION MAKING AT THE HEART OF SERVICE DELIVERY– YOU AS MANAGER?

Letter 1: What do healthcare managers do?

1 ILX Group. What is Prince? Available at: www.prince2.com/what-is-prince2.asp (accessed 3 December 2010).
2 JISC Infonet. Good Practice and Innovation – Change management. Available at: www.jiscinfonet.ac.uk/infokits/change-management (accessed 3 December 2010).

3   JISC Infonet. JISC Infokit – Change Management. Available at: www.jiscinfonet.ac.uk/
    infokits/change-management/printable-version.pdf (accessed 3 December 2010).
4   Office of Government Commerce. Skills and Competencies. Available at: www.ogc.
    gov.uk/delivery_lifecycle_skills_and_competencies.asp (accessed 3 December 2010).

Coffee break: what are your management roles and competencies?

1   NHS Knowledge and Skills Framework (NHSKSF) and The development review process
    (October 2004). Available at: www.dh.gov.uk/en/Publicationsandstatistics/Publications/
    PublicationsPolicyAndGuidance/DH_4090843 (accessed 3 December 2010).
2   Royal College of Nursing. NHS Knowledge and Skills Framework outlines for nurs-
    ing posts. RCN Guidance for nurses and managers in creating KSF outlines in the
    NHS 2005. Available at: www.rcn.org.uk/data/assets/pdf_file/0007/78667/002775.
    pdf (accessed 3 December 2010).
3   Royal College of Nursing. Agenda for Change. Available at: www.rcn.org.uk/agenda
    forchange (accessed 3 December 2010).
4   National Health Service. Graduate Management Training Scheme. Available at: www.
    nhsgraduates.co.uk (accessed 3 December 2010).

Letter 2: How do managers manage?

Coffee break: understanding people to manage people

Letter 3: Hit the ground running?

Coffee break: role continuity or change?

Letter 4: Decision making and change – reading the environment

1   Bible study tools. Ecclesiastes Chapter 9 (New International Version). Available at:
    www.biblestudytools.com/ecclesiastes/9.html (accessed 3 December 2010).

Coffee break: reading the environment

1   Department of Health. NHS Emergency planning guidance 2005. www.dh.gov.
    uk/en/Publicationsandstatistics/Publications/PublicationsPolicyAndGuidance/
    DH_4121072. (accessed 3 December 2010)
2   Department of Health. Emergency Planning. Available at: www.dh.gov.uk/en/
    Managingyourorganisation/Emergencyplanning/index.htm (accessed 3 December 2010).
3   Health and Safety Executive. Leading Health and Safety at Work. Available at: www.
    hse.gov.uk/leadership/index.htm (accessed 3 December 2010).

SECTION 3 DECISION MAKING AT THE POINT OF SERVICE DELIVERY

Letter 1: Managing processes – governance

1   CBC News. Air Transat fined $250,000 for air mistake. Available at: www.cbc.ca/
    canada/story/2001/09/06/airtransat010906.html (accessed 3 December 2010).

2 UK Parliament Hansard. Herald of Free Enterprise *HC Deb 24 July 1987 vol 120 cc677-95*. Available at: hansard.millbanksystems.com/commons/1987/jul/24/herald-of-free-enterprise (accessed 3 December 2010).

3 United States Consumer Product Safety Commission Washington DC 2027. Memorandum. June 7 2000. Available at: www.cpsc.gov/LIBRARY/Bedrail00.pdf (accessed 3 December 2010).

4 The Telegraph. Elderly patient died on trolley in understaffed hospital. Available at: www.telegraph.co.uk/news/uknews/1330512/Elderly-patient-died-on-trolley-in-understaffed-hospital.html (accessed 3 December 2010).

5 Nightingale F. Notes on Nursing. What it is and what it is not. 1860. http://digital.library.upenn.edu/women/nightingale/nursing/nursing.html#I (accessed 3 December 2010).

6 Care Quality Commission. Available at: www.cqc.org.uk (accessed 3 December 2010).

7 Care Quality Commission. Care Quality Commission enforcement policy Consultation. Available at: http://cpaa.org.uk/files/CQC_enforcement_policy_consultation_08.pdf (accessed 3 December 2010).

8 Health and Safety Executive. Health and safety regulation – a short guide 08/03. Available at: www.hse.gov.uk/pubns/hsc13.pdf (accessed 3 December 2010).

9 Health and Safety Executive. Health and safety legislation. Available at: www.hse.gov.uk/legislation/index.htm (accessed 3 December 2010).

10 Health and Safety Executive. COSHH Essentials, easy steps to control health risk from chemicals. Available at: www.coshh-essentials.org.uk/ (accessed 3 December 2010).

11 Health and Safety Executive. Five Steps to Risk Assessment. Available at: www.hse.gov.uk/risk/fivesteps.htm (accessed 3 December 2010).

12 Health and Safety Executive Riddor. Available at: www.hse.gov.uk/riddor/index.htm (accessed 3 December 2010).

Coffee break: managing processes—governance and risk reporting

1 Health and Safety Executive. Health and Safety Regulation A short guide. Available at: www.hse.gov.uk/pubns/hsc13.pdf pp. 5/7. (accessed 3 December 2010).

2 Health and Safety Executive. What is reportable? Available at: www.hse.gov.uk/riddor/guidance.htm#what (accessed 3 December 2010).

3 Health and Safety Executive. Heath and Safety at Work etc Act 1974. Available at: www.hse.gov.uk/legislation/hswa.htm (accessed 3 December 2010).

Letter 2: Governance and smart working processes

1 NHS Greater Glasgow and Clyde. Care Bundles. Available at: www.nhsggc.org.uk/CONTENT/default.asp?page=s1108 (accessed 3 December 2010).

2 Institute of Healthcare Improvement. What is a bundle? Available at: www.ihi.org/IHI/Topics/CriticalCare/IntensiveCare/ImprovementStories/WhatISABundle.htm (accessed 3 December 2010).

3 Mid Trent Critical care Network: Care Bundles. Available at: www.midtrentccn.nhs.uk/service-improvement/care-bundles (accessed 3 December 2010).

4 NHS Institute for innovation and improvement. The University of Warwick Going Lean in the NHS. Available at: www.institute.nhs.uk/option,com_joomcart/

Itemid,26/main_page,document__product_info/products_id,231.html (accessed 3 December 2010).

5   NHS Institute for Innovation and Improvement 2007. Going Lean in the NHS. www. institute.nhs.uk/option,com_joomcart/Itemid,26/main_page,document_product_info/products_id,231.html (accessed 3 December 2010).

6   NHS Institute for Innovation and Improvement. The productive ward module structure. Available at: www.institute.nhs.uk/quality_and_value/productivity_series/the_productive_ward_module_structure.html (accessed 3 December 2010).

Coffee break: governance, smart working processes and the business plan

1   Palmer C. Clinical governance: breathing new life into clinical audit. *Advances in Psychiatric Treatment*. 2002; 8: 470–76.

2   Department of Health. Clinical Governance. Available at: www.dh.gov.uk/en/Publichealth/Patientsafety/Clinicalgovernance/index.htm (accessed 3 December 2010).

3   Royal College of Nursing. Clinical Governance: an RCN resource guide. Available at: www.rcn.org.uk/_data/assets/pdf_file/0011/78581/002036.pdf. (accessed 3 December 2010).

4   Department of Health Government of Western Australia. Information series 1.1 Introduction to Clinical Governance. A Background paper. Available at: www.safetyandquality.health.wa.gov.au/docs/clinical_gov/Introduction_to_Clinical_Governance.pdf (accessed 3 December 2010).

Letter 3: Governance and workforce development

1   National Health Service. Healthcare Workforce Portal. Available at: www.healthcare-workforce.nhs.uk/index.html (accessed 3 December 2010).

Coffee break: intellectual and social capital

SECTION 4 DECISION MAKING AND RESOURCE MANAGEMENT

Letter 1: Governance and the staff journey: recognising the investment

1   Manchester Galleries. Available at: www.manchestergalleries.org/the-collections (accessed 3 December 2010).

2   Equality and Human Rights Commission. Available at: www.equalityhumanrights.com/ (accessed 3 December 2010).

3   The Bible New International Version, Proverbs 27: 23. Available at: http://Biblia.com (accessed 3 December 2010).

Coffee break: governance and management style

1   The Chartered Institute of Personnel and Development. Available at: www.cipd.co.uk/default.cipd (accessed 3 December 2010).

2   Advisory Conciliation and Arbitration Service. Available at: www.acas.org.uk/index.aspx?articleid=1461 (accessed 3 December 2010).

3   Computerweekly.com. Hospital sacks senior manager over stolen laptop. Available at: www.computerweekly.com/Articles/2008/08/12/231799/hospital-sacks-senior-manager-over-stolen-laptop.htm (accessed 3 December 2010).

4 Colchester Hospital NHS Trust. Press Release Disciplinary hearing 11 August 2008. Available at: www.colchesterhospital.nhs.uk/press_releases/pr_110808.pdf (accessed 3 December 2010).

5 Police in hospital deaths inquiry. Nurse dismissed after four patients die in intensive care unit. *The Independent,* 3 April 1996. Available at: www.independent.co.uk/news/police-in-hospital-deaths-inquiry-1302963.html (accessed 3 December 2010).

6 NHS Hampshire. Case studies of recent NHS Ffraud cases. Available at: www.hampshire.nhs.uk/component/content/article/53-ppsa/430-case-studies (accessed 3 December 2010).

Letter 2: Managing information and communication

1 Frimley Park Hospital NHS Trust Conflict of Interest and associated matters. Policy and Guidelines. August 2008.

Coffee break: freedom of information and communications strategy

1 Information Commissioner's Office. Available at: www.ico.gov.uk (accessed 3 December 2010).

2 Walsall Hospitals NHS Trust. Corporate Communications Strategy 2008-11. Available at: www.walsallhospitals.nhs.uk/Library/AboutUs/BoardPapers/May2008/ENC8corpommsstrategy8may2008.doc (accessed 3 December 2010).

Letter 3: Health informatics

1 British Computer Society: The Chartered Institute for IT. Available at: www.bcs.org/server.php?show=nav.9373 (accessed 3 December 2010).

2 The NHS Connecting for Health (2009). Learning to manage Health information: a theme for clinical education. Available at: www.connectingforhealth.nhs.uk/systemsandservices/capability/health/hidcurriculum/brochure.pdf (accessed 3 December 2010).

Coffee break: local procedures and information management

SECTION 5 DECISION MAKING AND THE SERVICE USER JOURNEY

Letter 1: The service user journey – health needs assessment

1 National Institute for Health and Clinical Excellence. Health needs assessment: A practical guide. Available at: www.nice.org.uk/aboutnice/whoweare/aboutthehda/hdapublications/health_needs_assessment_a_practical_guide.jsp (accessed 3 December 2010).

Coffee break: health needs assessment

1 National Institute for Health and Clinical Excellence. Health needs assessment: A practical guide. Available at: www.nice.org.uk/aboutnice/whoweare/aboutthe-hda/hdapublications/health_needs_assessment_a_practical_guide.jsp (accessed 3 December 2010).

2   Swansea's Health Social Care and Well-being (HSCWB) Needs Assessment (2007). Available at: www.healthchallengeswansea.org.uk/index.cfm?articleid=33111 (accessed 3 December 2010).

3   Association of Public Health Observatories. Available at: www.apho.org.uk (accessed 3 December 2010).

Letter 2: The service user journey – outcomes

1   Street, A. 2006 (Editorial) Future of quality measurement in the National Health Service Expert Review. *Pharmacoeconomics Outcomes Res.* 6 (3), pp. 245–248. Available at: www.york.ac.uk/media/che/documents/papers/che-2006-futurequality.pdf (accessed 3 December 2010).

2   Department of Health. High Quality Care for All: NHS next stage final report 2008. Available at: www.dh.gov.uk/en/Publicationsandstatistics/Publications/Publications PolicyAndGuidance/DH_085825 (accessed 3 December 2010).

3   Department of Health. High Quality Care for All (archived content). Available at: http://webarchive.nationalarchives.gov.uk/+/www.dh.gov.uk/en/Healthcare/High qualitycareforall/index.htm (accessed 3 December 2010).

4   HealthCare Commission. Available at: http://ratings2005.healthcarecommission. org.uk/Trust/Indicator/indicatorDescriptionShort.asp?indicatorId=1006 (accessed 3 December 2010).

Coffee break: knowing what to measure

1   Department of Health. Quality Accounts. Available at: www.dh.gov.uk/en/Healthcare/ Qualityaccounts/index.htm (accessed 3 December 2010).

SECTION 6 DECISION MAKING: WHERE IS IT ALL HEADING? STRATEGIC MANAGEMENT

Letter 1: Strategy: lost and found

Coffee break: not losing the way – strategic function

1   Department of Health (2003): Governing the NHS. A guide for NHS Boards. Available at: www.dh.gov.uk/en/Publicationsandstatistics/Publications/Publications PolicyAndGuidance/DH_4082638 (accessed 3 December 2010).

2   Dixon, A. and Alvarez-Rosete, A. Governing the NHS. Alternatives to an independent board. London, King's Fund; 2008. Available at: www.kingsfund.org.uk/research/ publications/governing_the.html (accessed 3 December 2010).

Letter 2: Where next?

Index

Coffee breaks in **BOLD**. Figures in *ITALIC*

Printed and bound by CPI Group (UK) Ltd, Croydon, CR0 4YY

23/10/2024

01777678-0013